CONCISE CLINICAL
EMBRYOLOGY

CONCISE CLINICAL EMBRYOLOGY
AN INTEGRATED, CASE-BASED APPROACH

Mark G. Torchia, DipBT, MSc, PhD

Associate Professor, Department of Surgery and Department of
Human Anatomy and Cell Sciences, Max Rady College of Medicine,
Rady Faculty of Health Sciences, University of Manitoba

Vice-Provost (Teaching and Learning), University of Manitoba

Winnipeg, Manitoba, Canada

T.V.N. (Vid) Persaud MD, PhD, DSc, FRCPath (Lond.), FAAA

Professor Emeritus and Former Head, Department of
Human Anatomy and Cell Science

Professor of Pediatrics and Child Health

Associate Professor of Obstetrics, Gynecology,
and Reproductive Sciences

Max Rady College of Medicine, Rady Faculty of Health Sciences,
University of Manitoba, Winnipeg, Manitoba, Canada

ELSEVIER

Elsevier
1600 John F. Kennedy Blvd.
Ste 1800
Philadelphia, PA 19103-2899

CONCISE CLINICAL EMBRYOLOGY:
AN INTEGRATED, CASE-BASED APPROACH

ISBN: 978-0-323-69615-9

Library of Congress Control Number: 2020951836

Content Strategist: Jeremy Bowes
Content Development Specialist: Erika Ninsin
Publishing Services Manager: Deepthi Unni
Project Manager: Srividhya Vidhyashankar
Design Direction: Margaret Reid

Printed in Canada

Last digit is the print number: 9 8 7 6 5 4 3 2 1

Preface

This comprehensive yet concise textbook is designed for students in all health fields learning human embryology, as well as for the review of human embryology in clinical practice. The text is copiously illustrated to provide visual cues and resources for better understanding. Accompanying this book, in online format, are 18 exceptional colour animations, with narrations, which will assist the student in learning the various stages of human embryo and fetal development.

A clinical case scenario is provided at the beginning of each chapter. These cases are not straightforward and many of the concepts or considerations will require the reader to seek information outside the direct field of clinical embryology; this helps to place the knowledge and details of embryology within the larger concept of clinical care. Follow-on scenarios for each case are found at the end of each chapter and provide the reader with an opportunity to further expand the ability to problem solve, think broadly and search for answers beyond this textbook. Answers are not provided to these cases so that they can be used for ongoing discussion amongst peers, advanced learning and knowledge testing.

Each chapter also provides fundamental molecular biology considerations. This information is derived from the extant literature and is based mainly on experiments with animal models including mice because the human cells or tissues required to examine such science are not generally available. As such, keep in mind that as knowledge of molecular genetics and biology progresses, the specific genes and their products that are identified may change or be expanded upon.

The section on Clinical Issues in each chapter provides a description of the common congenital anomalies and other clinical information related to the embryology details contained in the chapter. Finally, each chapter has a brief reference list that can be used to find additional details about the clinical cases, molecular biology and clinical embryology.

Learners wanting to test their knowledge or prepare for examinations will also benefit from the multiple choice questions we have provided through the website.

Acknowledgements

We are indebted to Mr. Jeremy Bowes, Senior Content Strategist, for his invaluable insights and unstinting support in the preparation of Concise Clinical Embryology. We are particularly grateful to Ms. Erika Ninsin, Content Development Specialist, Ms. Meghan Andress, Content Development Manager, and Ms. Sri Vidhya Vidhyashankar, Project Manager/Health Content Manager for their helpful suggestions. Finally, we would like to Dr. Brad Smith, University of Michigan, for graciously providing the image (Carnegie Stage 18 human embryo) which is on the cover of this book (Imaging performed at the Center for In-Vivo Microscopy, Duke University).

Contents

Video Table of Contents

SECTION 1

GENERAL DEVELOPMENT OF THE EMBRYO AND FETUS

1 Introduction

Case Scenario

A 26-year-old woman (GW) presents to you, a nurse practitioner at a public health clinic, with severe odynophagia. The history and physical examination leads you to strongly believe she has a streptococcal pharyngitis; a swab is taken for rapid strep test (which is positive) and you prescribe amoxicillin. When you inquire about her obvious pregnancy, GW reports being approximately 5 months pregnant based on when she remembered having had her last menstrual period. She said that the father is a 55-year-old companion. GW has been living on the street and in shelters for the past year since discharge from an inpatient facility for treatment of a crystal methamphetamine addiction. She vehemently denies use of methamphetamine since that treatment. She has not sought any other medical care in the interim. GW has had only one previous pregnancy which resulted in the birth of a son, now 5 years old, and currently living with the maternal grandparents. Her son was born with a bilateral cleft palate. You recommend a fetal ultrasound as soon as possible, to which she agrees.

Questions for reflection: Why might an ultrasound fetal assessment be warranted? What concerns might you have related to the health of GW? What impact, if any, might these issues have on the health of her fetus, including risk for anomalies? Is the father's age or the fact that her 5-year-old son had a cleft palate relevant to the current pregnancy? Why?

The study of embryology is essential for the understanding of both normal anatomy and congenital anomalies. Moreover, the practice of obstetrics and neonatal–perinatal medicine involves clinical embryology. Although infant mortality rates have been decreasing steadily in North America for the past 50 years, the 2018 rate in the United States remains at 5.6 per 1000 live births, 4.3 per 1000 in Canada and 11 per 1000 in Mexico. Given that congenital anomalies are the second leading cause of infant mortality (behind premature birth), the need to better understand the mechanisms of normal embryo and fetal development and the factors that impact this development, leading to congenital anomalies remains very high. The growing field of molecular biology and the development of many novel laboratory techniques have led to a significant improvement of our knowledge of the temporal and regional expression of genes and their products to control such processes as morphogenesis.

USING THIS TEXTBOOK

This textbook is designed to offer a concise knowledge base for the study or review of clinical embryology. The accompanying illustrations (drawing and medical imaging) provide a visual resource to further enhance the textual explanations and development paths.

A clinical case scenario is provided for each chapter. As you will discover, the cases are not straightforward, and many of the words, concepts or considerations will require the reader to seek information outside the direct field of clinical embryology—this helps to situate the knowledge and details of embryology within the larger concept of clinical care. The clinical case in this chapter is a good example. You will need to consider, for example, infectious disease, genetics, pharmacology and neonatal cardiology and combine that knowledge to answer the question. The follow-on scenarios to the original case, found at the end of each chapter, will further expand your need to problem solve, think broadly and search for answers beyond this textbook. Answers are not provided to the cases so that they can be used for ongoing discussion amongst peers, advanced learning and knowledge testing.

Each chapter also provides molecular biology considerations. This information is based mainly on experiments with animal models including mice because the human cells or tissues required to examine such science are not generally available. As such, keep in mind that as knowledge of molecular genetics and biology progresses, the specific genes and their products that are identified may change or be expanded upon.

Molecular Biology Considerations

- TFG-ß, BMP, FGF10, MX1, IRF6—most commonly implicated pathways for palatine clefting

The section Clinical Issues in each chapter provides a description of the common congenital anomalies and other clinical information, related to the embryology details contained in the chapter.

Finally, each chapter provides a brief reference list that can be used to find additional details about the clinical cases, molecular biology and details of clinical embryology. We encourage you to seek additional information during your studies as the timing of book printing, relative to the constant gain of knowledge and reporting, negates the possibility of including the very most recent literature, although the authors have tried their utmost to provide citations that are as current as possible.

OTHER IMPORTANT INFORMATION

Throughout this textbook, the specified age of embryos and fetuses as it relates to specific structures and other developments, has been quoted as fertilisation age—length of time from the date of fertilisation.

In the clinical context, gestational age is indicated as the time from the date of the start of the last menstrual period (LMP). Given that ovulation (and shortly thereafter, fertilisation) occurs typically around 14 days after the start of the menstrual period, gestational age LMP is approximately 2 weeks or 14 days greater than fertilisation age.

It is important to specifically describe the method used for indicating 'gestational age', so that confusion does not arise, especially when ordering or interpreting ultrasound images or comparing between times within a patient history.

Because the Federative International Committee on Anatomical Terminology does not recommend the use of eponyms, for the most part, this book follows suit (there are few exceptions to this when the clinical eponym is most commonly used).

There will be a number of terms in this book that may not be familiar to the reader, not limited to just those of embryology. It is recommended that the reader search for those definitions from a reliable source of such medical information.

Anatomical position and direction terms are used throughout this book. In adults, the terms anterior and posterior are used to describe the front and back of the body or limbs or relative positions of one structure to another. In the fetus or embryo, the terms ventral and dorsal are used, respectively. In addition, the terms caudal or rostral are used to denote a relationship to the head, whereas caudal is used to denote relationship to the caudal eminence or tail.

CLINICAL ISSUES

CLEFT PALATE

Palate clefts arise from failure of the lateral palatine process to fuse with:

- The primary palate (anterior palate cleft)
- Each other and the nasal septum (posterior palate cleft)

- The primary palate, with each other, and the nasal septum (secondary palate cleft).

Some clefts appear as part of single mutant gene or chromosomal syndromes or following the effects of teratogenic substances.

Case Outcome

Fetal ultrasound showed a male fetus of approximately 22 weeks of age (based on femur length, biparietal diameter, head circumference and abdominal circumference), which would approximately align with the predicted age based on the patient's last menstrual period. The ultrasound also detected an isolated membranous ventricular septal defect (VSD). The remainder of the examination was normal. Sixteen weeks later, GW had a vaginal delivery. The neonate had good Apgar scores (7/8 at 1/5 minutes). The birth weight was at the 4th percentile. Otherwise the infant appeared normal.

Additional reflection: What is the error rate for estimating delivery dates from a single ultrasound examination at 22 weeks? Was it likely that the ultrasound was in error or that GW delivered early or both or neither? Why? What is the likely cause of the VSD? How common are these anomalies and what treatment is required and when, if any? What might be the causes for the baby to be born at such a low percentile birth weight? What other concerns might you have regarding the health of the neonate or GW?

BIBLIOGRAPHY

Methods for estimating the due date. Committee Opinion No. 700. American College of Obstetricians and Gynecologists. Obstet Gynecol 2017;129:e150–154.

Deshpande AS, Goudy SL. Cellular and molecular mechanisms of cleft palate development. Laryngoscope Investig Otolaryngol 2019;4(1):160–4.

2 Reproductive Organs and Gametogenesis

Case Scenario

A 24-year-old woman (KR) presents at her new family physician with difficulty conceiving. She and her husband have been trying to have a child for almost 5 years. Her husband recently had his sperm count and morphology tested, and this has proven to be normal. KR is now seeking additional advice and investigation for herself. KR describes her menstrual cycle as varying in length, and occasionally she has missed her period entirely. Otherwise, she has been healthy. KR also has severe acne. It had been previously controlled after a course of antibiotics and topical gel treatment when she was 21 years old, but the acne has now returned. KR mentioned that she has had acne since she was 13 years old. Recently, she began to notice more dark hair growth on her chin and areolas, and that her leg hair has had a noticeable regrowth after shaving. Her body mass index (BMI) is 20.6.

Questions for reflection: Are there other fertility considerations for KR's husband beyond the semen analysis that might be investigated? What might be the connection, if any, between KR's recurrent acne and potential fertility concerns? What further testing or consultation might be appropriate for KR?

PUBERTY

The reproductive organs (or primary sex characteristics) develop in utero. Maturation of the reproductive organs and the appearance of secondary sex characteristics (such as breast growth, presence of axillary and public hair) occur after puberty—the transitional process from childhood to adulthood. The exact biological trigger that starts the process of puberty is unclear; however the initiation of gonadotropin-releasing hormone (GnRH) pulsing leads to the secretion of luteinising hormone (LH) and follicle-stimulating hormone (FSH) by the pituitary. LH and FSH, in turn, stimulate the secretion of androgens and oestrogens from the gonads (the hypothalamic–pituitary–gonadal axis). The Tanner scale or sexual maturity rating (SMR; 1 = preadolescence to 5 = sexual maturity) is used as a framework on which to objectively classify the development of secondary sexual characteristics.

In females, the appearance of breast buds is the start of SMR 2, the first indication of the onset of puberty, and typically occurs between the ages of 8 and 12 years. Simultaneously, the labia, uterus and ovaries increase in size, and the tissues of the uterus and vagina (endometrium and mucosa, respectively) increase in thickness. It is not until approximately 30 months later that menstruation begins, although the regularity of menstruation may be variable for a number of months as anovulatory cycles are common. In general, the age at which puberty begins in females has been decreasing since the mid-1940s; the reasons for this are not known, but may be related to the increase in child obesity or other environmental factors.

In males, the enlargement of the testicles and development of pubic hair are the early signs of the onset of puberty, typically occurring at approximately 10 years of age (SMR 2). The testes and the penis continue to enlarge until late adolescence under the influence of both LH and testosterone secretion as do the prostate and seminal vesicles. Sperm appear approximately 3 to 4 years following the onset of puberty. Although males undergo some degree of breast enlargement, gynaecomastia, during puberty, this tends to resolve spontaneously in later stages of adolescence.

MALE REPRODUCTIVE ORGANS

The penis (Fig. 2.1) acts as the conduit for both urine and ejaculate to exit the body. It consists of the glans or head, which in uncircumcised men is covered by the prepuce or foreskin. The urethral opening is found at the tip of glans penis which forms from the expanded distal end of the corpus spongiosum. The vascular corpus cavernous surrounds the corpus spongiosum, which when expanded by blood, provide the erectile function of the penis. The erectile tissue of the corpus spongiosum supports the urethra and maintains its patency during an erection.

The testes are the oval-shaped, sperm- and testosterone-producing organs found within the scrotum. The testes are covered with a thick fibrous capsule, the tunica albuginea, and contain a series of coiled seminiferous tubules within which sperm development occurs. The seminiferous tubules are connected to the tubuli recti. The rete testes are connected to the epididymis. The duct of the epididymis (ductus deferens) passes from the epididymis through the inguinal canal into the pelvic cavity. The ductus deferens traverses the prostate gland where it joins the urethra. The prostate gland secretes prostatic fluid into the semen, which supports transportation and nutrition of the sperm. Paired seminal vesicles and the bulbourethral glands provide additional secretion to the semen.

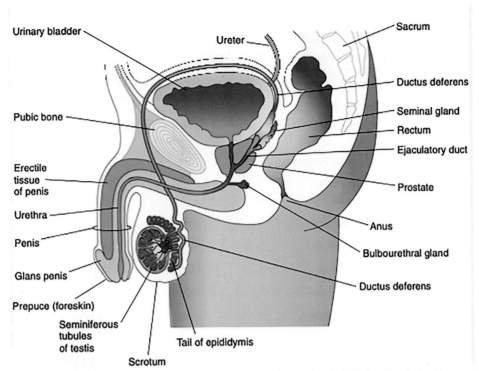

Fig. 2.1 Sagittal section of the male pelvic region. (From Moore KL, Persaud TVN, & Torchia MG. *The Developing Human: Clinically Oriented Embryology.* 10th ed. Philadelphia: Elsevier; 2015.)

FEMALE REPRODUCTIVE ORGANS

The vagina (Fig. 2.2) is a fibromuscular organ that extends from the external genitalia (vulvar structures) to the cervix of the uterus. The opening of the vagina is situated posterior to the opening of the urethra and is covered by the labia minora. The uterus is a thick-walled muscular organ consisting of the body (upper two-thirds) and the cervix (lower one-third). The cervix is cylindrical with constricted opening at both ends, the internal and external os. The body of the uterus is comprised of three tissue layers, endometrium (internal), myometrium (middle muscular) and perimetrium (external). The endometrium can be further distinguished into the compact, spongy and basal layers, and varies in thickness according to stages of the menstrual cycle.

The uterine tubes are continuous with the uterine horns found at the superior end of the uterus, the fundus. The uterine tubes are approximately 10-cm long, and consist of four parts: infundibulum, ampulla, isthmus and uterine part. The tubes are lined with cilia that help to propel the ovum and sperm, first to the site of fertilisation (ampulla) and then to assist in moving the cleaving zygote to the uterus for implantation.

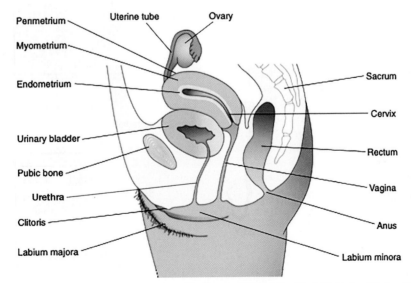

Fig. 2.2 Sagittal section of the female pelvic region. (From Moore KL, Persaud TVN, & Torchia, MG. *Before We Are Born: Essentials of Embryology and Birth Defects.* 9th ed. Philadelphia: Elsevier; 2016.)

The ovaries are oval-shaped glands adjacent to the uterus and the uterine tube infundibulum, with its finger-like fimbriae. The ovaries produce the oocytes, as well hormones (oestrogen and progesterone) that regulate the process of sexual development, menstruation and pregnancy.

The external female genitalia consist of the labia minora, labia majora and the clitoris.

GAMETOGENESIS

Gametogenesis (oogenesis and spermatogenesis) (Fig. 2.3) is the process that produces oocytes and sperms from bipotential primordial germ cells and prepares these gametes for fertilisation. The sperm and oocyte are highly specialised

NORMAL GAMETOGENESIS

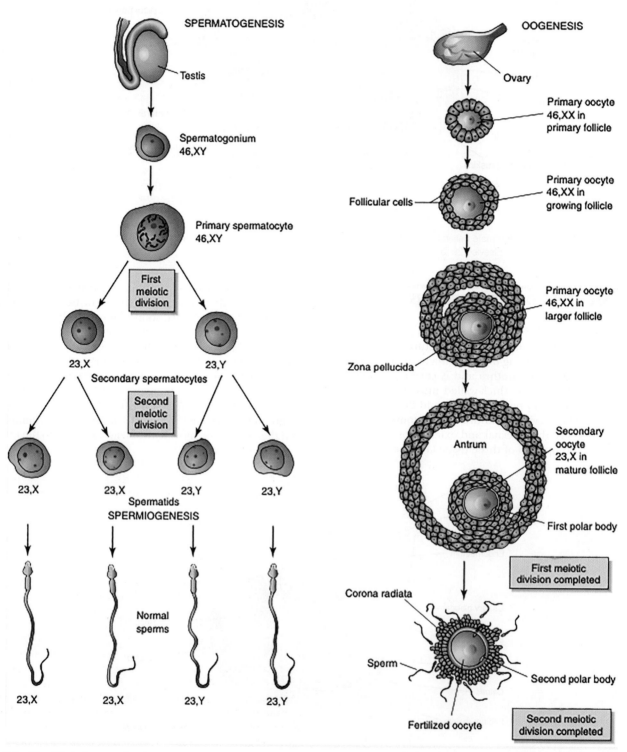

Fig. 2.3 Simplified diagram showing normal gametogenesis. (From Moore KL, Persaud TVN, & Torchia MG. *The Developing Human: Clinically Oriented Embryology.* 10th ed. Philadelphia: Elsevier; 2015.)

sex cells, each of which contains the haploid number of chromosomes that are present in somatic cells. The number of chromosomes is reduced during meiosis, a special type of cell division that occurs only during gametogenesis. Meiosis involves two meiotic cell divisions resulting in diploid germ cells giving rise to haploid gametes.

The first meiotic division is a reduction division because the chromosome number is reduced to haploid by pairing of homologous chromosomes in prophase and their segregation at anaphase with one representative of each pair randomly going to each pole of the meiotic spindle. At this stage, the chromosomes are double-chromatid chromosomes. (The X and Y chromosomes are not homologues, but they have homologous segments at the tips of their short arms and pair in these regions only.) This disjunction of paired homologous chromosomes is the physical basis of segregation, the separation of allelic genes during meiosis. The second meiotic division does not have an interphase, but each double-chromatid chromosome divides, and each half, or chromatid, is drawn to a different pole. Thus the haploid number of chromosomes remains, and each daughter cell has one representative of each chromosome pair (now a single-chromatid chromosome). The process of meiosis provides constancy of the chromosome number from generation to generation, allows random assortment of maternal and paternal chromosomes between the gametes and relocates segments of maternal and paternal chromosomes by crossing over of chromosome segments, which produces a recombination of genetic material.

SPERM CHARACTERISTICS AND DEVELOPMENT

Sperms are highly differentiated, actively motile cells consisting of a head and a tail (Fig. 2.4) and approximately 4 μm in length. The head forms most of the bulk of the sperm and contains the nucleus. The anterior two-thirds of the head is covered by the acrosome, a saccular organelle

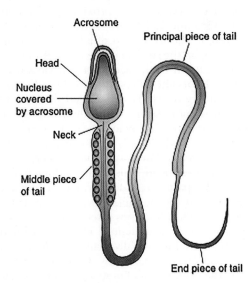

Fig. 2.4 Main parts of the human sperm. (From Moore KL, Persaud TVN, & Torchia MG. *The Developing Human: Clinically Oriented Embryology.* 10th ed. Philadelphia: Elsevier; 2015; Fig. 2.5.)

containing several enzymes and other factors which, when released, facilitate dispersion of the follicular cells of the corona radiata and sperm penetration of the zona pellucida during fertilisation. The tail has four segments: the connecting, middle, principal and end pieces, and it provides the motility of the sperm for transport to the site of fertilisation. The axoneme is the motility machinery of the sperm and is comprised of cytoskeleton and dyneins (ATPase molecular motors). The helically arranged mitochondria in the middle piece provide the energy required for motility. Sperm travel at approximately 3 mm/min.

Spermatogonia (primordial male germ cells) are dormant in the seminiferous tubules of the testes during the fetal and postnatal periods. At puberty, spermatogenesis begins, a 2-month highly complex process that transforms spermatogonia into mature sperms. More than one dozen different subtypes of male germ cells have been identified. There are also a number of cells and factors within the testes involved in sperm development. Peritubular myoid cells are found surrounding and supporting the seminiferous tubules and are thought to regulate Sertoli cells, assist in managing the blood–testis barrier (an important controller of the germ cell microenvironment) and push testicular fluid with sperm towards the rete testis. Leydig cells (LCs) are found clustered near seminiferous tubules and the adjacent blood vessels. LCs produce testosterone, which is released into the systemic circulation. LCs ensure a much higher local concentration of testosterone, which is required for normal sperm production. LCs also produce oestradiol from testosterone, which appears to be required for successful spermatogenesis. Sertoli cells (SCs) make up approximately 20% of the epithelial cells of the seminiferous tubules. The role of the SCs is complex and broad. Their unique structure allows each SC to shepherd up to 50 germ cells during differentiation; this is accomplished by sophisticated cytoskeletal elements. SCs produce anti-Müllerian hormone, critical to the normal embryological develop of male and female reproductive organs. SCs also act as macrophages, and produce inhibin B (regulating FSH production) and androgen-binding protein.

The male germ cells are arranged in the seminiferous tubules in a specific manner with least-mature cells in the basal compartment and more-mature cells found adjacent to the lumen.

The earliest germ cells in the testes (gonocytes) remain in G0 phase of the cell cycle until after birth. In the first few neonatal months, they are transformed into inactive spermatogonia which begin to undergo rapid mitosis at approximately 6 years of age. Later, at puberty, the spermatogonia undergo the process of spermatogenesis. Briefly, spermatogonia first develop into primary spermatocytes, the largest germ cells in the seminiferous tubules of the testes. Each primary spermatocyte subsequently undergoes the first meiotic division to form two haploid secondary spermatocytes. These secondary spermatocytes undergo the second meiotic division and form four haploid spermatids. The spermatids are gradually transformed into four mature sperms by a process known as spermiogenesis. When spermiogenesis is complete, the sperms enter the lumina of the seminiferous tubules. Sperms are transported passively from the seminiferous tubules to the epididymis, where they are stored.

OOCYTE CHARACTERISTICS AND DEVELOPMENT

The mature (secondary) oocyte (Fig. 2.5) is an immotile cell with a diameter of approximately 100 μm, making it one of the largest cells in the female human body, and just visible to the unaided eye. It typically contains a transparent moderately granular cytoplasm with refractile structures such as lipid, lipofuscin bodies, and autophagic vacuoles. A single polar body is also associated with the secondary oocyte (see later).

Oogenesis transforms oogonia (primordial female germ cells) into mature oocytes. All oogonia develop prenatally, and the process of oogenesis ceases following menopause. In early fetal life, oogonia proliferate by mitosis and enlarge to form primary oocytes, each surrounded by a single layer of flattened, connective tissue follicular cells. The primary oocyte enclosed by this layer of follicular cells constitutes a primordial follicle. As the primary oocyte enlarges during puberty, the follicular epithelial cells become columnar shaped and the oocyte becomes covered with the glycoproteinaceous zona pellucida. Primary oocytes begin the first meiotic divisions before birth, but completion of prophase does not occur until puberty. The follicular cells surrounding the primary oocytes secrete a substance, oocyte maturation inhibitor, which keeps the meiotic process of the oocyte arrested. With puberty, the ovarian follicle (typically only one) matures each month. As a follicle matures, the primary oocyte increases in size and shortly before ovulation it completes the first meiotic division to give rise to a secondary oocyte and the first polar body. The secondary oocyte receives almost all the cytoplasm; the polar body is destined for degeneration. At ovulation, the nucleus of the secondary oocyte begins the second meiotic division, but it

progresses only to metaphase. If a sperm penetrates the secondary oocyte at fertilisation, the second meiotic division is completed, and most cytoplasm is again retained by one cell, the fertilised oocyte. The second polar body is formed and will degenerate.

There are approximately 2 million primary oocytes in the ovaries of a neonate, but most of them regress during childhood so that by adolescence no more than about 40,000 primary oocytes remain. Of these, only approximately 400 become secondary oocytes and are expelled at ovulation during the reproductive period. Very few of these oocytes, if any, are fertilised. The long duration of the first meiotic division (up to 45 years) may account in part for the relatively high frequency of meiotic errors that occur with increasing maternal age.

FEMALE REPRODUCTIVE CYCLE

The female reproductive cycle (Fig. 2.6) is highly complex and involves activities of the hypothalamus, pituitary gland, ovaries, uterus, uterine tubes, vagina and mammary glands, all towards preparation of the reproductive system for pregnancy.

GnRH secreted by the hypothalamus stimulates the anterior lobe of the pituitary gland to release FSH, which stimulates the development of ovarian follicles and the production of oestrogen by the follicular cells, and LH, which triggers ovulation and stimulates follicular cells and corpus luteum to produce progesterone and causes growth of the follicles and endometrium.

As the primary follicle increases in size, the adjacent connective tissue organises into a capsule, the theca folliculi. This theca soon differentiates an internal vascular and glandular layer (theca interna) and a capsule-like layer (theca externa). The follicular cells produce a stratified layer around the oocyte. Fluid-filled spaces appear around the follicular cells, which coalesce to form the antrum, containing follicular fluid at this stage; the ovarian follicle is then called a secondary follicle. The primary oocyte is pushed to one side of the follicle. At approximately the midpoint of the cycle, FHS and LH stimulation cause rapid follicle growth leading to the formation of a small avascular spot, follicular stigma, on the surface of the ovary. Rupture of the stigma and expulsion of the secondary oocyte (ovulation) occurs 12 to 24 hours after this surge of LH production. The expelled secondary oocyte is surrounded by the zona pellucida and one or more layers of radially arranged follicular cells (corona radiata). Shortly after ovulation, the walls of the ovarian follicle and theca folliculi collapse and develop into the corpus luteum. The corpus luteum secretes progesterone and some oestrogen, causing the endometrial glands to secrete and prepare the endometrium for implantation of the blastocyst. If the oocyte is fertilised, the corpus luteum enlarges to form a corpus luteum of pregnancy and increases its hormone production. The corpus luteum of pregnancy remains functionally active throughout about the first 20 weeks of pregnancy. By this time, the placenta has assumed the production of oestrogen and progesterone necessary for the maintenance of pregnancy. If the oocyte is not fertilised, the corpus luteum involutes and degenerates 10 to 12 days after ovulation.

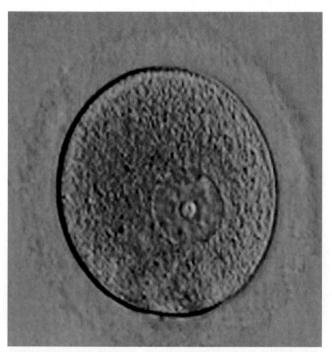

Fig. 2.5 Photomicrograph of a human oocyte. (From Zhang P, Zucchelli M, Bruce S, et al. Transcriptome profiling of human pre-implantation development. PLoS One 2009; 4(11): e7844. With permission.)

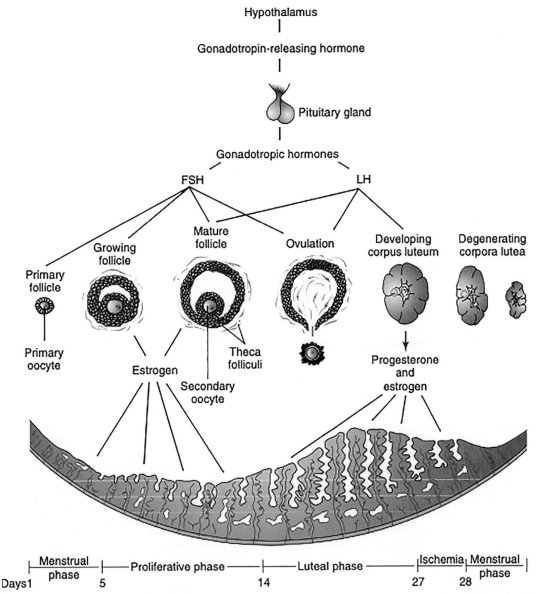

Fig. 2.6 Schematic drawing of the ovarian and menstrual cycles. (From Moore KL, Persaud TVN, & Torchia MG. *The Developing Human: Clinically Oriented Embryology.* 10th ed. Philadelphia: Elsevier; 2015.)

MENSTRUAL CYCLE

Changes in the oestrogen and progesterone levels cause cyclic changes in the structure of the female reproductive tract, notably the uterine endometrium (Fig. 2.6). The menstrual cycle is a continuous process lasting on average 28 days, with each phase gradually passing into the next. Day 1 is designated as the day menstrual flow begins. In the menstrual phase (4–5 days), the functional layer of the endometrium is sloughed off as the menses (blood discharged from the vagina combined with small pieces of endometrial tissue). After menstruation, the remaining endometrium is thin.

During the proliferative phase (9 days), the ovarian follicles grow and the uterine surface epithelium reforms and covers the endometrium. The uterine glands increase in number and length and endometrial spiral arteries elongate. The luteal (secretory) phase lasts approximately 13 days and coincides with the formation, functioning and growth of the corpus luteum. The progesterone produced by the corpus luteum stimulates the glandular epithelium to secrete a glycogen-rich material. The glands become wide, tortuous and saccular, and the endometrium thickens because of the influence of progesterone and oestrogen from the corpus luteum. As the spiral arteries grow into the superficial compact layer, they become increasingly coiled. The venous network becomes complex, and large lacunae (venous spaces) develop in the endometrium. If fertilisation does not occur the corpus luteum degenerates, oestrogen and progesterone levels fall, and the secretory endometrium enters an ischemic phase. The spiral arteries constrict, glandular secretion stops, interstitial fluid is reduced, endometrium shrinks and venous stasis occurs. This leads to patchy ischaemic necrosis of the functional layer of the endometrium. Rupture of damaged vessel walls allows blood to leak into the surrounding connective tissue, resulting in bleeding (typical loss of 20–80 mL).

If fertilisation occurs, the zygote undergoes cleavage and blastogenesis, and the blastocyst begins to implant in the endometrium (sixth day of the luteal phase). The embryo syncytiotrophoblast produces chorionic gonadotropin, which keeps the corpora luteum secreting oestrogens and progesterone; the luteal phase continues and menstruation does not occur.

Molecular Biology Considerations

- PI3K/PTEN and TSC/mTOR pathways—activation of primordial follicles
- GDF9 and BMP15—development of secondary and pre-ovulatory follicle
- cAMP meiotic arrest
- MAPK3/1—ovulation control
- bFGF—maintenance of blood–testis barrier
- TGF-a/b and GNDF—maintenance of spermatogenesis microenvironment
- PModS—regulates Sertoli cell function
- HOX—shaping of sperm head

CLINICAL ISSUES

FERTILITY

In 85% to 90% of cases, heterosexual couples are able to achieve pregnancy through sexual intercourse. In the remaining couples, fertility issues for both the male and female require investigation; these male/female concerns often coexist. In men, the most common causes of reduced fertility are a blockage of sperm delivery, altered sperm morphology, motility and function and reduced sperm numbers. Previous infection, retrograde ejaculation, prior trauma and tumours are examples of causes of blocked semen flow. Abnormal sperm morphology includes large or double heads and bent or double tails; causes include genetic disorders, exposure to environmental toxins or high testicular temperatures. Men with fewer than 10 million sperms per millilitre of semen are less likely to be fertile, especially when the specimen contains immotile and abnormal sperms. Environmental factors (drug or alcohol abuse, exposure to environmental toxins), medication and hormone imbalance are only a few of the reasons that low sperm counts may occur.

In women, the most common causes of infertility are blockage of oocyte transportation attributed to tubal scarring or endometriosis, reduced production of oocytes because of increased age, and hormonal imbalances such as from polycystic ovarian syndrome (PCOS) and obesity.

CONTRACEPTION

The use of hormonal methods of female contraception can result in some or all of thickened cervical mucus, alteration of the endometrium, prevention of ovulation or blockage of sperm. These contraceptives include progestin-only pills, combined oestrogen–progestin pills, emergency contraceptive pills, vaginal rings, contraceptive patches and injectable long-acting medications including drug-integrated implants. Intrauterine devices may contain either hormones or copper and prevent sperm from reaching the ovum or

implantation. No hormone-based contraceptive is available for men. Barrier methods, including condoms (male or female) and contraceptive diaphragms, prevent sperm from entering the vagina or uterus, respectively. Sterilisation (implant, vasectomy or tubal ligation) are permanent forms of birth control.

NONDISJUNCTION

Nondisjunction is an error in cell division in which there is failure of a chromosomal pair (autosome or sex chromosome) to separate during mitosis or meiosis, resulting in numeric aberrations of chromosomes. Nondisjunction may occur during maternal or paternal gametogenesis, resulting in some gametes having 24 chromosomes while others have only 22. If these gametes should become fertilised with a normal gamete, a zygote with either trisomy (three copies of a chromosome) or monosomy (one copy of a chromosome) results. Clinical conditions resulting from such nondisjunction include trisomy 21 (Down syndrome), trisomy 18 (Edwards syndrome), XXY trisomy (Klinefelter syndrome) and monosomy X (Turner syndrome).

Case Outcome

KR was sent for blood tests as well as endocrine and gynaecological consultations. Higher than normal levels of androgens were detected in her blood; there were no other abnormal findings. A pelvic examination was normal. A pelvic ultrasound demonstrated multiple cysts on her ovaries (see Fig. 2.7). She was diagnosed with polycystic ovarian syndrome (PCOS) and returned to her family physician for discussion of treatment options and follow-up.

Additional reflection: Did KR present with the typical signs for PCOS? Given KR's desire for children, how might this be a consideration for her long-term treatment of PCOS? What is the likelihood of KR conceiving a child, should her husband's fertility prove to be normal? What might be some psychological implications of PCOS?

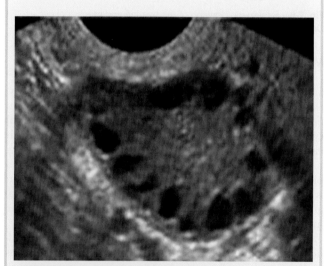

Fig. 2.7 Pelvic ultrasound demonstrating cystic structures on the oval in polycystic ovarium syndrome. (From Karakas SE. New biomarkers for diagnosis and management of polycystic ovary syndrome. Clin Chim Acta 2017; 471: 248–253. With permission.)

QUESTIONS

1. Which of the following types of germ cell does not undergo cell division?
   a. spermatogonia
   b. primary oocytes
   c. spermatids
   d. secondary spermatocytes
   e. oogonia

2. An infant is diagnosed as having 47 chromosomes instead of 46. This abnormal condition (trisomy) results from:
   a. gene mutation
   b. nondisjunction
   c. disturbances in spermiogenesis
   d. disturbances in mitosis
   e. abnormal spermatogonia

BIBLIOGRAPHY

Datta J, Palmer MJ, Tanton C, et al. Prevalence of infertility and help seeking among 15,000 women and men. Hum Reprod 2016;31:2108–18.

Neto FTL, Bach PV, Najari BB, Li PS, Goldstein M. Spermatogenesis in humans and its affecting factors. Sem Cell Dev Biol 2016;59:10–26.

Pasquali R. Contemporary approaches to the management of polycystic ovary syndrome. Ther Adv Endocrinol Metb 2018;9(4):123–34.

3 Fertilisation and Reproductive Technologies

Case Scenario

A 49-year-old woman (PG) presents to her family physician reporting a positive home pregnancy test and claims to be approximately 2-months pregnant based on timing of her last normal menstrual period. She is concerned because this is her first pregnancy; she and her partner have not used birth control for the past three months because her menstrual periods have been very irregular for the past year and she believed that she was 'in menopause and not infertile'.

A second pregnancy test was ordered which was positive. An ultrasound (endovaginal sonogram) showed a live embryo with crown–rump length of approximately 9 mm, aged between 35 and 38 days.

Given PG's age, she was counselled regarding the options for (or no) prenatal screening for fetal aneuploidies.

Questions for reflection: Why is PG's age a concern and how may age impact normal gametogenesis. What types of prenatal screening are available and at what gestational age? Which of the tests is considered diagnostic? What are the most common aneuploidies?

FERTILISATION

During ovulation, the fimbriated end of the uterine tube becomes closely applied to the surface of the ovary. The sweeping action of the tube and of fluid currents produced by the ciliated mucosal cells of the fimbriae, causes the extruded oocyte to enter the infundibulum of the uterine tube. The oocyte then passes into the ampulla of the tube, mainly as the result of tube peristalsis. During sexual intercourse and ejaculation, sperms are rapidly transported from the epididymis to the urethra by peristaltic contractions of the thick muscular coat of the ductus deferens. Between 200 and 600 million sperms are deposited in the vagina, around the external os and the fornix, and then some pass through the cervical canal. The cervical mucus increases in amount and becomes less viscid during ovulation, making it more favourable for sperm passage. Approximately 200 sperms reach the ampulla of the uterine tube; the remainder degenerate and are absorbed in the female genital tract. Sperms must undergo capacitation, lasting approximately 7 hours, before they are able to fertilise the oocyte. During this process, a glycoprotein coat and seminal proteins are removed from the surface of the sperm acrosome and the membrane components of the sperms are extensively altered. Sperms are usually capacitated while they are in the uterus or uterine tubes by substances secreted by these parts of the female genital tract. Oocytes are usually fertilised within 12 hours of ovulation, and it appears that they cannot be fertilised after 24 hours (see Video 3.1).

The usual site of fertilisation is in the ampulla of the uterine tube. If the oocyte is not fertilised, it slowly passes along the tube to the body of the uterus, where it degenerates and is resorbed.

Fertilisation is a sequence of coordinated events (Fig. 3.2), beginning with the passage of a sperm through the corona radiata. Hyaluronidase released from the sperm acrosome, tubal mucosa enzymes and sperm motion appear to cause dispersal of the follicular cells of the corona radiata. Passage of a sperm through the zona pellucida is the next phase and also results from the action of enzymes released from the acrosome, including acrosin, esterase and neuraminidase. Once a sperm penetrates the zona pellucida, a change in the properties of the zona pellucida (zona reaction) occurs that makes it impermeable to other sperms. The zona reaction is believed to result from the action of lysosomal enzymes released by cortical granules near the plasma membrane of the oocyte. The contents of these granules also cause changes in the plasma membrane that make it impermeable to other sperms. Fusion and localised breakdown of cell membranes of the oocyte and sperm occurs next, resulting in the head and tail of the sperm entering the cytoplasm of the oocyte (the cell membrane and mitochondria of the sperm remain behind). Penetration of the oocyte by a sperm activates the oocyte into completing the second meiotic division and forming a mature oocyte and a second polar body. The maternal chromosomes decondense and the nucleus of the mature oocyte becomes the female pronucleus.

The nucleus of the sperm enlarges to form the male pronucleus and the tail of the sperm degenerates. Both pronuclei duplicate their DNA and the oocyte becomes an ootid. When the pronuclei fuse into a single diploid aggregation of chromosomes, the ootid becomes a zygote. The chromosomes in the zygote become arranged on a cleavage spindle in preparation for cleavage of the zygote. The zygote is genetically unique.

CLEAVAGE OF THE ZYGOTE AND FORMATION OF THE BLASTOCYST

Cleavage occurs approximately 30 hours after fertilisation as the zygote, within the zona pellucida, passes along the uterine tube towards the uterus. Cleavage consists of repeated mitotic divisions of the zygote, resulting in a rapid increase in the number of cells (blastomeres) and decrease

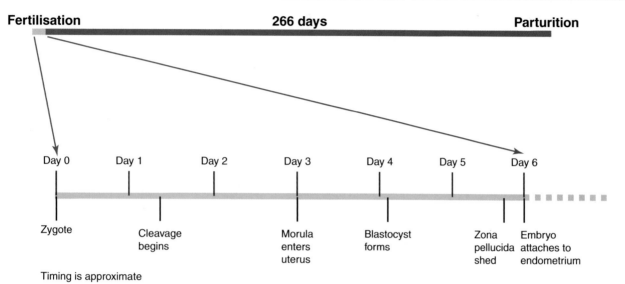

Fig. 3.1   Timeline of development related to fertilisation.

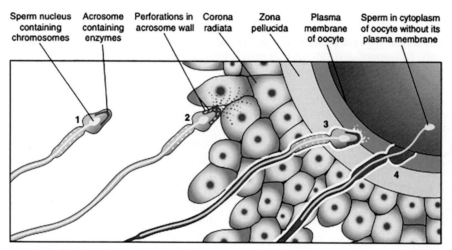

Fig. 3.2   Events taking place in fertilisation. (From Moore KL, Persaud TVN, & Torchia MG *The Developing Human: Clinically Oriented Embryology.* 10th ed. Philadelphia: Elsevier; 2015.)

in the size of subsequent blastomeres with each successive cleavage division. After the nine-cell stage, the blastomeres undergo compaction, changing their shape and tightly aligning themselves against each other to form a compact ball of cells. Compaction changes the cell cytoskeleton, permitting greater cell-to-cell interaction. Polarisation of the blastomeres into apical and basolateral domains also takes place. Compaction is necessary for segregation of the internal cells that will form the embryoblast (inner cell mass) of the blastocyst from surrounding cells that form the trophoblast (Fig. 3.3). At the 12- to 32-blastomeres stage, the developing embryo is called a morula. Shortly after the morula enters the uterus (approximately 4 days postfertilisation), the fluid-filled blastocystic cavity appears inside the morula separating the blastomeres into the trophoblast (thin outer cell layer giving rise to the embryonic part of the placenta) and the embryoblast (centrally located blastomeres which form the embryo). Early pregnancy factor (EPF), an immunosuppressant protein, is secreted by the trophoblastic cells and aids in the prevention of early maternal immune attack of the embryo (see Video 3.2).

After the blastocyst has floated in the uterine secretions for approximately 2 days, shedding of the zona pellucida occurs, permitting the blastocyst to increase rapidly in size. While in the uterus, the embryo derives nourishment from secretions of the uterine glands. At approximately 6 days, the blastocyst (usually adjacent to the embryonic pole) attaches to the endometrial epithelium. The trophoblast proliferates rapidly and differentiates into two layers—an inner layer of cytotrophoblast that is mitotically active and forms new mononuclear cells that migrate into the increasing mass of syncytiotrophoblast, and an outer layer of syncytiotrophoblast (multinucleated protoplasmic mass) (Fig. 3.4). The syncytiotrophoblast begins to invade the uterine connective tissue so that the blastocyst can now derive its nourishment from the eroded maternal tissues. Endometrial cells assist to control the depth of penetration of the syncytiotrophoblast. At approximately 7 days, a layer of cells, the hypoblast (primary endoderm), appears on the surface of the embryoblast facing the blastocystic cavity. Comparative embryological data suggest that the hypoblast arises by delamination of blastomeres from the embryoblast.

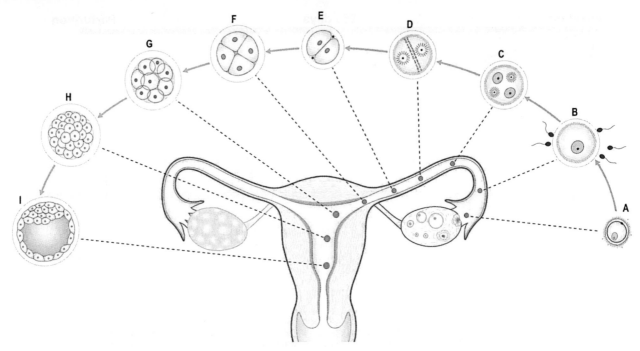

Fig. 3.3 Stages of development during the first week. (A) Ovulated oocyte; (B) fertilisation; (C) pronuclei formation; (D) first cleavage spindle; (E–G) cleavage of zygote; (H) morula; (I) blastocyst. (From Mitchell B, Sharma R. *Embryology: An Illustrated Colour Text.* 2nd ed. London: Elsevier; 2009.)

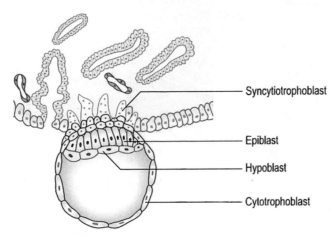

Fig. 3.4 A 7-day blastocyst beginning to implant. (From Mitchell B, Sharma R. *Embryology: An Illustrated Colour Text.* 2nd ed. London: Elsevier; 2009.)

Molecular Biology Considerations

- SPAM1, HYAL5, ACE3, ADAMS1–3—gamete fusion
- Hippo—segregation of embryoblast from trophoblast
- TGF-b—proliferation and differentiation of the trophoblast

CLINICAL ISSUES

ASSISTED REPRODUCTIVE TECHNOLOGIES

IN VITRO FERTILISATION AND EMBRYO TRANSFER

In vitro fertilisation (IVF) of oocytes and transfer of cleaving zygotes into the uterus have provided an opportunity for many women who are sterile to have children. Since 1978, when Robert G. Edwards and Patrick Steptoe pioneered IVF, several million children have been born following an IVF procedure. The steps involved during IVF and embryo transfer are briefly noted. Beginning on day 1 of the menstrual cycle, ovarian follicles are stimulated to grow and mature (superovulation), typically by the administration of a drug that increases follicle-stimulating hormone (FSH) and/or luteinising hormone (LH) secretion by the pituitary. At the optimal time (often determined by ultrasound), another medication (synthetic human chorionic gonadotropin [hCG]) is given to trigger ovulation. Using an ultrasonically guided, minimally invasive procedure, several mature oocytes (typically 8–15) are aspirated from mature ovarian follicles. The oocytes are then placed in a Petri dish containing a special culture medium and capacitated sperms. Fertilisation of the oocytes and cleavage of the zygotes are monitored by microscope for 3 to 5 days. Depending on the mother's age, one to three of the resulting embryos (four-cell to eight-cell stage, or early blastocysts) are transferred by introducing a catheter through the vagina and cervical canal into the uterus. Any remaining embryos are frozen for later use. Approximately 2 weeks later, a pregnancy test is performed.

CRYOPRESERVATION OF EMBRYOS

Early embryos resulting from IVF can be preserved for long periods by freezing them in liquid nitrogen with a cryoprotectant (e.g., glycerol or dimethyl sulfoxide). Successful transfer of four- to eight-cell embryos and blastocysts to the uterus after thawing is now a common practice. The longest period of sperm cryopreservation that resulted in a live birth was reported to be 21 years.

INTRACYTOPLASMIC SPERM INJECTION

A sperm can be injected directly into the cytoplasm of a mature oocyte. This technique has been successfully used for the treatment of couples in whom typical IVF has failed, or in cases where there are too few sperms available.

ASSISTED IN VIVO FERTILISATION

Gamete intrafallopian (intratubal) transfer enables fertilisation to occur in the uterine tube. It involves superovulation (similar to that used for IVF), oocyte retrieval, sperm collection and laparoscopic placement of several oocytes and sperms into the uterine tubes. Using this technique, fertilisation occurs in the ampulla, its usual location.

SURROGATE MOTHERS

Some women produce mature oocytes but are unable to become pregnant, for example, a woman who has had a hysterectomy. In these cases, IVF may be performed, and the embryos transferred to another woman's uterus for fetal development and delivery.

PREGNANCY TESTING

Most pregnancy tests are based on the detection or measurement of human chorionic gonadotropin (hCG) produced by the syncytiotrophoblast. hCG can be measured in urine or in blood. hCG rapidly increases in concentration from the time of early implantation (approximately day 6–12). The blood testing performed by clinical laboratories uses a more sensitive assay, and it also measures hCG concentration which can be followed over time depending on clinical needs. There are a number of biological and pharmacological factors that can produce false positive and negative hCG test results including heterotrophic antibodies, rheumatoid factors and ectopic pregnancies.

Transvaginal ultrasonography can detect the gestational sac at approximately 2.5 to 3 weeks following conception.

ANEUPLOIDY

Aneuploidy, usually resulting from nondisjunction, is any deviation from the diploid number of 46 chromosomes and is the most common (3%–4% of pregnancies) and clinically significant numeric chromosomal abnormalities.

MONOSOMY X

The incidence of Turner syndrome (45,X) is about 1:8000 live births. Only 1% of monosomy X female embryos survive, with 45,X being the most common abnormality detected in all spontaneous abortions. When it is possible to trace, it is the paternal X chromosome that is missing in approximately 75% of cases. In some cases, mosaicism occurs (XX/X and XY/X mosaics) and in these cases there is a lesser degree of abnormalities. The abnormalities typically seen with 45,X include small stature, ovarian dysgenesis, broad chest with wide-spaced nipples, congenital lymphedema and a short and/or webbed neck.

AUTOSOMAL TRISOMY

Trisomy is the most common aneuploidy. Trisomy of autosomes is mainly associated with three syndromes: trisomy 18 (Edwards syndrome, 1.3:10,000 live births), trisomy 13 (Patau syndrome, 0.8:10,000) and trisomy 21 (Down syndrome, 12:10,000). Infants with trisomy 13 and trisomy 18 are severely malformed (trisomy 13—includes defects of the lip,

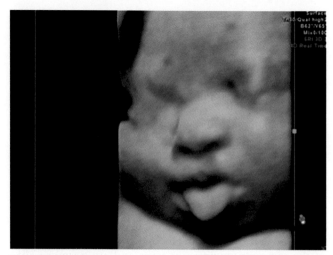

Fig. 3.5 Three-dimensional ultrasound image of a fetus with trisomy 21, showing characteristic features including a protruding tongue (macroglossia).

nose and eyes, holoprosencephaly, polydactyly, skin defects; trisomy 18—includes clenched hands, prominent occiput, short sternum, small pelvis, cryptorchidism) and have major neurodevelopmental disabilities. Infants with these life-limiting disorders (trisomy 18 and 23) have a 1-year survival rate of approximately 6% to 12%. Infants with trisomy 21 (Fig. 3.5) have abnormalities that include cognitive deficiency, hypotonia, bradycephaly, upward slanting palpebral fissures, protruding tongue, small ears, heart defects such as endocardial defects, ventricular septal defect or atrial septal defect, and a transverse palmar flexion crease. More than one-half of trisomic embryos spontaneously abort early. Trisomy of the autosomes occurs with increasing frequency as maternal age increases. For example, trisomy 21 occurs once in approximately 1400 births among mothers between the ages of 20 and 24 years but once in approximately 25 births among mothers 45 years and older. Because of the current trend of increasing maternal age, it has been estimated that children born to women older than 34 years will account for 39% of infants with trisomy 21.

TRISOMY OF SEX CHROMOSOMES

These disorders are not usually detected until puberty because there are no characteristic physical findings in infants or children. These disorders include XYY syndrome (1:1000; tall stature, cognitive disabilities, severe acne, autism spectrum disorder, normal fertility), XXX (1:1000; normal puberty, normal fertility, some degree of cognitive deficiency can occur); and XXY syndrome (Klinefelter syndrome) (1:500; most common cause of hypogonadism and infertility, gynaecomastia, inadequate virilisation, long limbs and possible developmental delay).

MOSAICISM

A person with at least two cell lines with two or more genotypes is considered a mosaic. The autosomes or sex chromosomes may be involved. The defects usually are less serious than in persons with monosomy or trisomy. For instance, the features of Turner syndrome are not as evident in 45,X/46,XX mosaic females as in the usual 45,X females.

Although mosaicism usually results from nondisjunction, it can also occur through the loss of a chromosome by anaphase lagging; chromosomes separate normally, but one of them is delayed in its migration and is eventually lost.

MULTIPLE GESTATIONS

In North America, twins naturally occur approximately once in every 85 pregnancies, triplets approximately once in 90^2 pregnancies, quadruplets once in 90^3 pregnancies and quintuplets approximately once in every 90^4 pregnancies. Twins that originate from two zygotes are dizygotic (DZ) twins whereas twins that originate from one zygote are monozygotic (MZ) twins. Two-thirds of twins are DZ, with marked racial differences whereas the incidence of MZ twinning is approximately the same in all populations. DZ twins may be of the same sex or different sexes and are no more alike genetically than brothers or sisters born at different times. The fetal membranes and placentas vary according to the origin of the twins. DZ twins always have two amnions and two chorions, but the chorions and placentas may be fused. Anastomoses between blood vessels of fused placentas of DZ twins may result in erythrocyte mosaicism. MZ twins are genetically identical; physical differences between MZ twins are caused by environmental differences, chance variation and uneven X-chromosome activation. MZ twinning usually results from division of the embryoblast into two embryonic primordia, with each embryo in its own amniotic sac but sharing the same chorionic sac and placenta (monochorionic–diamniotic twin). Uncommonly, early separation of embryonic blastomeres (e.g., during the two-cell to eight-cell stages) results in MZ twins with two amnions, two chorions and two placentas that may or may not be fused. Twin transfusion syndrome occurs in as many as 10% to 15% of monochorionic–diamniotic MZ twins. There is shunting of arterial blood from one twin through unidirectional umbilical–placental arteriovenous anastomoses into the venous circulation of the other twin. The donor twin is small, pale and anaemic whereas the recipient twin is large and has polycythaemia. In lethal cases, death results from anaemia in the donor twin and congestive heart failure in the recipient twin. Late division of early embryonic cells, such as division of the embryonic disc during the second week, results in MZ twins that are in one amniotic sac and one chorionic sac. A monochorionic–monoamniotic twin placenta is associated with fetal mortality rates that are higher by up to 10%, with the cause being cord entanglement. Because ultrasonographic studies are a common part of prenatal care, it is known that early death and resorption of one member of a twin pair is common. Triplets may be derived from one zygote and be identical, two zygotes and consist of identical twins and a singleton or three zygotes and be of the same sex or of different sexes. The determination of twin zygosity is done by molecular diagnosis.

PREIMPLANTATION GENETICS

In couples with inherited genetic disorders and using IVF, preimplantation genetic diagnosis can determine the genotype of the embryo and allow selection of a chromosomally healthy embryo for transfer. Preimplantation genetic diagnosis can be carried out 3 to 5 days after IVF of the oocyte. One or two cells (blastomeres) are removed from the embryo and these cells are then analysed before transfer into the uterus. The sex of the embryo can also be determined from one blastomere taken from a six- to eight-cell dividing zygote, and analysed by polymerase chain reaction and fluorescence in situ hybridisation techniques. This procedure has been used to detect female embryos during IVF in cases in which a male embryo would be at risk of a serious X-linked disorder. The polar body may also be tested for diseases where the mother is the carrier (Fig. 2.15A).

Case Outcome

Patient PG opted for noninvasive prenatal testing (NIPT) through cell-free DNA (cfDNA) screening. This testing was conducted approximately 3 weeks after her previous visit (8 weeks post conception—10 weeks gestational age). The test results demonstrated a high risk for trisomy 21 (Down syndrome).

A diagnostic chorionic villus sampling (CVS) was then performed that confirmed the diagnosis of trisomy 21. PG opted to continue the pregnancy. A later fetal ultrasound demonstrated enhanced nuchal translucency (Fig. 3.6), but no cardiovascular anomalies. The remainder of the pregnancy was uneventful, and PG delivered a baby girl at 38 weeks.

Additional reflection: What is the difference between a screening test and a diagnostic test? How is CVS performed, at what gestational age, and with what possible risks to fetus and the mother? What is a nuchal translucency, and why was there a concern about cardiovascular anomalies?

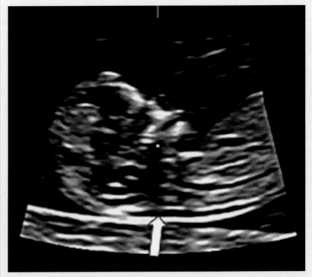

Fig. 3.6 Ultrasound of a fetus demonstrating an enhanced nuchal translucency *(arrow)*.

QUESTIONS

1. How many sperms would probably be deposited by a normal young adult male in the vagina during intercourse:
   a. 300,000
   b. 3 million
   c. 30 million
   d. 300 million
   e. 3 billion

2. The secondary oocyte completes the second meiotic division:
   a. before ovulation
   b. during ovulation
   c. at fertilisation
   d. before birth
   e. at puberty

3. The sperm penetrates the zona pellucida, partially assisted by enzymes that are released from which portion of the sperm:
   a. middle piece
   b. acrosome
   c. neck
   d. main piece
   e. head

4. Morphologically abnormal sperm may cause:
   a. monosomy
   b. congenital anomalies
   c. trisomy
   d. abnormal embryos
   e. infertility

BIBLIOGRAPHY

Jelin AC, Sagasser KG, Wilkins L. Prenatal genetic testing options. Pediatr Clin North Am 2019;66:281–93.

Bamberg C, Hecher K. Update on twin-to-twin transfusion syndrome. Best Pract Res Clin Obstet Gynaecol 2019;58:55–65.

Katz DJ, Teloken P, Shoshany O. Male infertility – The other side of the equation. Aust Fam Physician 2017;46:641–6.

4 Implantation and Week 2

Case Scenario

A 32-year-old woman, having had two previous successful pregnancies, presented to her family physician with unusually heavy menstruation. Her last normal menstrual period was exactly 2 months ago. She previously had a very regular cycle and normal menstrual flow. She did not complain of any abdominal pain. She has been on oral contraception for the past 3 years and felt that she had been compliant.

On physical examination, there was mild tenderness in her lower abdomen. Her blood pressure and heart rate were normal. Her haemoglobin level and white cell count were normal. Vaginal examination did not reveal any causes of bleeding although her posterior fornix was tender on digital examination. A pregnancy test was positive and an ultrasound examination in the office revealed an empty uterine cavity and fluid present in the rectouterine pouch (Fig. 4.1).

She was sent immediately to the nearby hospital for further care and treatment.

Questions for reflection: How could the pregnancy test be positive yet the woman is menstruating? Similarly, how could she be pregnant yet the uterine cavity is empty? What kind of fluid might be in the rectouterine pouch? What is your diagnosis and why? What further testing might be important?

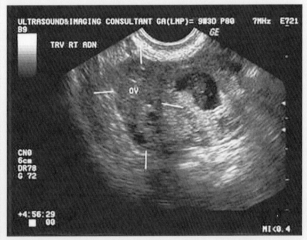

Fig. 4.1 Ultrasound image as per case.

IMPLANTATION

The mechanisms of implantation involve synchronisation between the invading blastocyst and a prepared endometrium. The window of implantation is relatively brief, 2 to 3 days, and occurs during a restricted time period, 6 to 10 days after ovulation and fertilisation—the mid-secretory stage of the menstrual cycle. At this time, and under the influence of progesterone and oestrogen, the cellular features of the endometrium are altered; pinopods (microvilli) form on the epithelial cells, cellular vacuoles move towards the apical end of cells, the uterine connective tissue is more oedematous, and some of the connective tissue cells accumulate large quantities of glycogen and lipids and expand in size, becoming the decidual cells (see Video 4.1).

The syncytiotrophoblast and the blastocyst slowly implant in the endometrium. Syncytiotrophoblastic cells displace endometrial cells at the implantation site, reach the basement membrane and then extend invadopodia between the cells, leading to degradation of the extracellular matrix. This invasion allows the syncytiotrophoblast to reach the vascular connective tissues and blood vessels. The syncytiotrophoblast engulfs decidual cells to provide embryonic nutrition. Some endometrial cells undergo apoptosis which facilitates the invasion. Endometrial cell signalling also helps to modulate the depth of penetration of the syncytiotrophoblast. The blastocyst is completely embedded by day 8 to 10. Initially the entry location is covered with fibrin after which endometrial cells proliferate to cover the implantation site.

Individual lacunae (Fig. 4.2) soon appear in the syncytiotrophoblast. These become filled with a mixture of maternal blood from the ruptured endometrial capillaries and cellular debris of eroded uterine glands, providing nutritive material to the embryo. Communication of the eroded endometrial capillaries with the lacunae in the syncytiotrophoblast establishes the earliest uteroplacental circulation. Oxygenated blood passes into the lacunae from the spiral endometrial arteries and poorly oxygenated blood is removed from them through the endometrial veins.

In a 12-day embryo, adjacent syncytiotrophoblastic lacunae have fused to form lacunar networks, the primordia of the intervillous spaces of the placenta. The endometrial capillaries around the implanted embryo become congested and dilated to form maternal sinusoids, thin-walled terminal vessels that are larger than ordinary capillaries. The syncytiotrophoblast erodes the sinusoids, and maternal blood flows freely into the lacunar networks. The trophoblast absorbs nutritive fluid from the lacunar networks, which is transferred to the embryo.

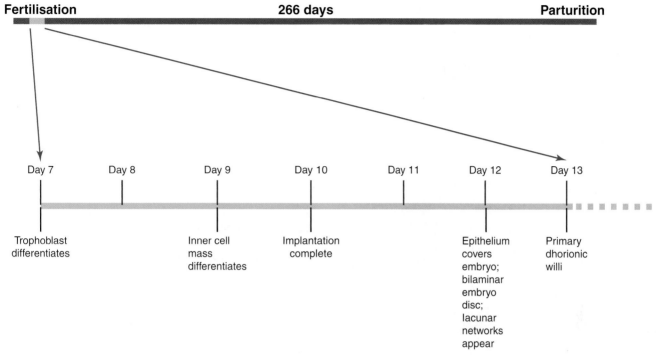

Timing is approximate

Fig. 4.2 Timeline of development related to implantation and week 2 of development.

BILAMINAR EMBRYO

As implantation of the blastocyst progresses, the primordium of the amniotic cavity appears in the embryoblast. Amniogenic cells, amnioblasts, separate from the epiblast and form the amnion, which encloses the amniotic cavity. Concurrently, morphological changes occur in the embryoblast resulting in a flat, almost circular embryonic disc, which is bilaminar (Fig. 4.3), consisting of the:

- epiblast—the thicker layer of high columnar cells related to the amniotic cavity; and
- hypoblast—the thinner layer of small cuboidal cells adjacent to the exocoelomic cavity.

The pluripotent epiblast forms the floor of the amniotic cavity and is continuous peripherally with the amnion. The hypoblast forms the roof of the exocoelomic cavity and is continuous with the thin exocoelomic membrane (Fig. 4.3). The exocoelomic membrane, together with the hypoblast, lines the primary umbilical vesicle. The bilaminar embryonic disc now lies between the amniotic cavity and umbilical vesicle. Cells from the umbilical vesicle endoderm form a layer of connective tissue, the extraembryonic mesoderm which surrounds the amnion and umbilical vesicle. The extraembryonic mesoderm increases and isolated coelomic spaces appear within it which rapidly fuse to form the extraembryonic coelom surrounding the amnion and umbilical vesicle (except where they are attached to the chorion by the connecting stalk). As the extraembryonic coelom forms, the primary umbilical vesicle decreases in size and a smaller secondary

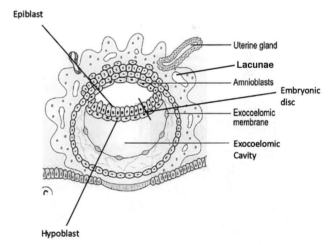

Fig. 4.3 Implanted blastocyst at 12 days. (Modified from Mitchell B, Sharma R. *Embryology: An Illustrated Colour Text.* 2nd ed. London: Elsevier; 2009.)

umbilical vesicle forms. This smaller vesicle is formed by extraembryonic endodermal cells that migrate from the hypoblast inside the primary umbilical vesicle.

DEVELOPMENT OF CHORIONIC SAC

The end of the second week is characterised by the appearance of primary chorionic villi (Fig. 4.4), that form columns with syncytial coverings. These cellular extensions grow into the syncytiotrophoblast forming primary chorionic villi, the

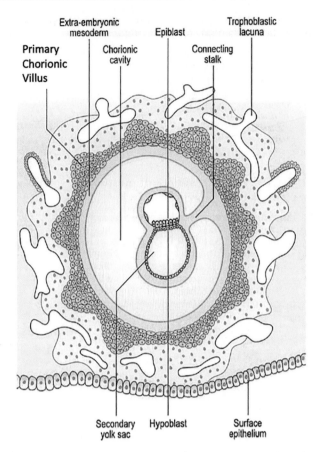

Fig. 4.4 Implanted embryo at 13 days. (Modified from Mitchell B, Sharma R. *Embryology: An Illustrated Colour Text.* 2nd ed. London: Elsevier; 2009.)

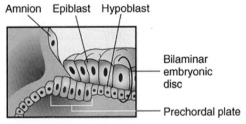

Fig. 4.5 Details of the prechordal plate. (Modified from Moore KL, Persaud TVN, & Torchia MG. *The Developing Human: Clinically Oriented Embryology.* 10th ed. Philadelphia: Elsevier; 2015.)

first stage in the development of the chorionic villi of the placenta.

The extraembryonic coelom splits the extraembryonic mesoderm into two layers: the extraembryonic somatic mesoderm, lining the trophoblast and covering the amnion and the extraembryonic splanchnic mesoderm, surrounding the umbilical vesicle (Fig. 4.4). The extraembryonic somatic mesoderm and the two layers of trophoblast form the chorion (wall of the chorionic sac). The embryo, amniotic sac and umbilical vesicle are suspended in the chorionic sac by the connecting stalk. At 14 days, the hypoblastic cells in a discrete area of the embryonic disc become columnar and form the prechordal plate (Fig. 4.5); the site of the primordial mouth. The prechordal plate serves as a signalling centre for controlling development of cranial structures, including the forebrain and eyes.

Molecular Biology Considerations

- MUC1, integrins (e.g., α1β1, HB-EGF)—implantation (maternal factors)
- Wnt—endometrial receptivity
- L-selectin—apposition of blastocyst to endometrium (blastocyst factor)
- Cx43—angiogenesis at implantation site
- miRs—communication between blastocyst and endometrium (blastocyst derived)

CLINICAL ISSUES

INHIBITION OF IMPLANTATION

The administration of progestins or antiprogestins (morning-after pills, a type of emergency contraceptive) for several days beginning shortly after unprotected sexual intercourse, inhibits ovulation and may also inhibit implantation of the blastocyst. An intrauterine device (IUD) usually interferes with implantation by causing a local uterine inflammatory reaction. An IUD is typically a primary contraceptive but may also be used for emergency contraception, by preventing fertilisation. Some IUDs contain progesterone, which is slowly released and interferes with the development of the endometrium so that implantation does not usually occur. Other IUDs have a wrap of copper wire. Copper is directly toxic to sperms and also causes uterine endothelial cells to produce substances that are toxic to sperms.

ECTOPIC IMPLANTATION

Implantation of blastocysts usually occurs in the superior part of the body of the uterus.

However, blastocysts sometimes implant outside the uterus (ectopia). Between 95% to 98% of ectopic implantations occur in the uterine tubes, most often in the ampulla and isthmus. The incidence of ectopic pregnancy ranges from 1 in 80 to 1 in 250 pregnancies, depending on many factors. In the United States, the frequency of ectopic pregnancy is approximately 2% of all pregnancies and rupture of a tubal pregnancy is responsible for about 3% of pregnancy-related deaths.

A woman with a tubal pregnancy has signs and symptoms of pregnancy but may also have abdominal pain and tenderness because of distention of the uterine tube, abnormal bleeding and pelvic peritonitis. The pain may be confused with appendicitis if the pregnancy is in the right uterine tube. Ectopic pregnancies produce β human chorionic gonadotropin (hCG) at a slower rate than normal pregnancies so pregnancy testing may give false-negative results if performed too early.

Transvaginal ultrasonography is extremely helpful in the early detection of ectopic tubal pregnancies.

There are several causes of tubal pregnancy, often related to factors that delay or prevent transport of the cleaving zygote into the uterus. Such factors include mucosal adhesions in the uterine tube or from blockage of the tube caused by scarring resulting from pelvic inflammatory disease. Unruptured tubal pregnancies may be managed medically (intramuscular methotrexate) and/or surgically (laparoscopic salpingotomy or salpingectomy) depending on the circumstances. Ectopic tubal pregnancies may result in rupture of the uterine tube and haemorrhage into the peritoneal cavity, followed by death of the embryo. Tubal rupture and haemorrhage are emergencies and a salpingectomy is performed.

When blastocysts implant in the isthmus of the uterine tube, the tube tends to rupture earlier because this narrow part of the tube is relatively inflexible, and there is often extensive bleeding. When blastocysts implant in the uterine (intramural) part of the tube they may develop beyond 8 weeks before rupture occurs.

Blastocysts that implant in the ampulla or on the fimbriae of the uterine tube may be expelled into the peritoneal cavity, where they can implant in the rectouterine pouch. In exceptional cases, an abdominal pregnancy may continue to full term and the fetus may be delivered alive through a laparotomy. Usually, however, the placenta attaches to the peritoneum or abdominal organs which causes considerable intraperitoneal bleeding. An abdominal pregnancy very significantly increases the risk of maternal death from haemorrhage.

In rare cases of cervical implantations, the placenta becomes firmly attached to fibrous and muscular tissues of the cervix, often resulting in bleeding, which requires subsequent surgical intervention, such as hysterectomy.

GESTATIONAL TROPHOBLASTIC DISEASES

Molar pregnancies (1:1500 pregnancies), a type of gestational trophoblastic disease (GTD), are classified as either complete or partial. The main mechanisms for development of complete hydatidiform moles include fertilisation of an oocyte with an absent or inactive pronucleus followed by duplication (monospermic mole) or fertilisation of an empty oocyte by two sperms (dispermic mole). Most complete hydatidiform moles are monospermic, the genetic origin of the nuclear DNA is paternal, and an embryo is absent but trophoblastic proliferation continues following implantation. This proliferation produces excessively elevated levels of hCG. A partial hydatidiform mole usually results from fertilisation of a normal oocyte by two sperms—dispermy. Most women with molar pregnancies present with significant vomiting, vaginal bleeding, enlarging uterus and a failed pregnancy. Ultrasound can detect the delayed spontaneous abortion or anembryonic pregnancy. Molar pregnancies are most often treated by suction curettage followed by anti-D prophylaxis.

Most hydatidiform moles are not cancerous. However some develop into invasive moles, which are locally invasive and nonmetastatic. In less than 5% of molar pregnancies, a choriocarcinoma develops. Choriocarcinomas are highly metastatic and can spread rapidly through the lymphatic vessels or bloodstream to various sites such as the lungs, vagina, liver, bone, intestine and brain. Chemotherapy is the treatment option of choice and, depending on the degree of metastases, radiation therapy and/or surgery may also be considered. These tumours can occur even following treatment of a molar pregnancy, which is why follow-up testing of hCG is important to ensure that hCG falls back to normal levels, indicating successful treatment of the molar pregnancy.

Case Outcome

The patient underwent a transvaginal ultrasound examination in hospital confirming a left tubal pregnancy with likely hemoperitoneum. Later that day, a diagnostic laparoscopy was performed. Hemoperitoneum was confirmed resulting from a bleeding left tubal pregnancy in the area of the ampulla. All other structures were normal. A left salpingectomy was performed with peritoneal lavage. The patient was discharged 24 hours later.

Additional reflection: Did this patient exhibit the typical presentation for tubal pregnancy? Is the rate of tubal pregnancy changing and, if so, what might be some reasons?

QUESTIONS

1. The wall of the chorionic sac is composed of:
   a. cytotrophoblast and syncytiotrophoblast
   b. two layers of trophoblast lined by extraembryonic somatic mesoderm
   c. trophoblast and the exocoelomic membrane
   d. two layers of trophoblast and extraembryonic splanchnic mesoderm
   e. amniotic sac and the umbilical vesicle

2. The amniotic cavity if found between the trophoblast and the:
   a. extraembryonic mesoderm
   b. inner cell mass
   c. exocoelomic membrane
   d. connecting stalk
   e. chorion

3. The most common location for an ectopic pregnancy is:
   a. on the ovary
   b. in the peritoneal cavity
   c. in the superior cervix
   d. in the isthmus of the uterine tube
   e. in the ampulla of the uterine tube

4. Which of the following is correct as it relates to gestational trophoblastic diseases:
   a. Most complete hydatidiform moles are monospermic
   b. Most partial hydatidiform moles are typically monospermic
   c. There is continued growth of the embryo although the trophoblast undergoes involution
   d. Unless treated immediately, most hydatidiform moles become choriocarcinomas
   e. In most cases, women with hydatidiform moles are asymptomatic

BIBLIOGRAPHY

Committee on Practice Bulletins – Gynecology. Practice Bulletin No. 193. Tubal Ectopic Pregnancy. American College of Obstetrics and Gynecology; 2018.

Cuman C, Van Sinderen M, Gantier MP, et al. Human blastocyst secreted microRNA regulate endometrial epithelial cell adhesion. EBioMedicine 2015;2:1528–35.

Fukui Y, Hirota Y, Matsuo M, et al. Uterine receptivity, embryo attachment, and embryo invasion: Multistep processes in embryo implantation. Reprod Med Biol 2019;18:234–40.

Su R-W, Fazleabas AT. Implantation and establishment of pregnancy in human and nonhuman primates. Adv Anat Embryol Cell Biol 2015;216:189–213.

Weeks 3 to 8—General Organogenesis

Case Scenario

A 47-year-old woman (JM) presented to her family physician with heavy menstrual bleeding and abdominal cramping. She was concerned because bleeding during her period is usually lighter, and there were more clots than she had seen previously. Also, the timing of her periods had been erratic over the past few months and she was concerned that she might have cancer; her mother had died at age 55 years of ovarian cancer. JM reported no other symptoms. Her past obstetric history was nulligravida. She is sexually active. Physical examination was normal (blood pressure 118/76 mmHg, heart rate 78 beats per minute, respiratory rate 17 breaths per minute, temperature 36.8° C) except for slight distention of the abdomen and very mild lower pelvic tenderness. Moderate active bleeding was noted during pelvic examination. The cervix was open; there was no cervical or adnexal tenderness. Haematology, blood chemistry and urinalysis were all within normal limits.

Questions for reflection: Might JM be approaching menopause? How would this be clinically evaluated? What diagnostic tests might be appropriate for her? Why? Are the JM symptoms typical for ovarian cancer? What other diagnoses might be considered?

GASTRULATION

Gastrulation is the beginning of morphogenesis (development of body form) and is the most significant event occurring during the third week. During gastrulation the bilaminar embryonic disc is converted into a trilaminar embryonic; the three germ layers develop, which are precursors of all embryonic tissues. At the same time, the axial orientation of the embryo is established. Extensive cell shape changes, rearrangement, movement and alterations in adhesive properties contribute to the process of gastrulation. Each of the three germ layers (ectoderm, mesoderm and endoderm) gives rise to specific tissues and organs. For instance, embryonic ectoderm gives rise to the epidermis, central and peripheral nervous systems, eyes and internal ears, neural crest cells, and many connective tissues of the head. Embryonic endoderm is the source of the epithelial linings of the respiratory and alimentary (digestive) tracts, including the glands opening into the gastrointestinal tract and glandular cells of associated organs such as the liver and pancreas. Embryonic mesoderm gives rise to all skeletal muscles, blood cells, the lining of blood vessels, all visceral smooth muscular coats, serosal linings of all body cavities, ducts and organs of the reproductive and excretory

systems and most of the cardiovascular system. Excluding the head and limbs, mesoderm is the source of all connective tissues, including cartilage, bones, tendons, ligaments, dermis and stroma (connective tissue) of internal organs (see Video 5.1).

The first morphological sign of gastrulation is the formation of the primitive streak on the dorsal surface of the epiblast of the bilaminar embryonic disc. By the beginning of the third week, this thickened linear band of epiblast (Fig. 5.2) appears caudally in the median plane of the embryonic disc and results from the proliferation and movement of cells of the epiblast to the median plane of the embryonic disc. The appearance of the primitive streak delineates craniocaudal axis, cranial and caudal ends, dorsal and ventral surfaces, and right and left sides of the embryo. As the streak elongates by addition of cells to its caudal end, the cranial end proliferates to form the primitive node. Concurrently, a narrow furrow, the primitive groove, develops in the primitive streak that is continuous with a small depression in the primitive node, the primitive pit. The primitive groove and pit result from the invagination of epiblastic cells. Later, cells leave the deep surface of the primitive streak (Fig. 5.3) and form mesenchyme – a connective tissue consisting of small, spindle-shaped cells loosely arranged in an extracellular matrix of sparse collagen fibres. Some mesenchyme forms mesoblast (undifferentiated mesoderm), which produces intraembryonic mesoderm. The primitive streak actively forms mesoderm until the early part of the fourth week; thereafter, production of mesoderm slows down. Cells from the epiblast, as well as from the primitive node and other parts of the primitive streak, displace the hypoblast, forming embryonic endoderm in the roof of the umbilical vesicle. The cells remaining in the epiblast create the embryonic ectoderm.

Caudal to the primitive streak, the cloacal membrane indicates the future site of the anus. The embryonic disc remains bilaminar here because the embryonic ectoderm and endoderm are fused. The primitive streak undergoes regressive changes and disappears by the end of the fourth week.

NOTOCHORD

Mesodermal cells migrate cranially from the primitive node and pit to form a median cord, the notochordal process (Fig. 5.4), which then develops a lumen, the notochordal canal. The notochordal process grows in a cranial direction in between the ectoderm and endoderm until it reaches

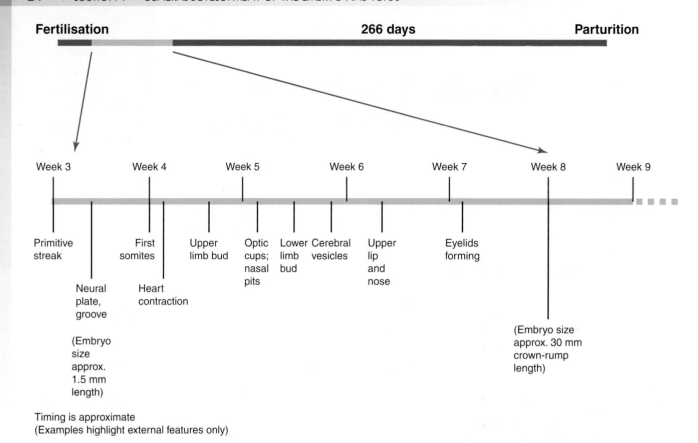

Timing is approximate
(Examples highlight external features only)

Fig. 5.1 Timeline of development related to general organogenesis.

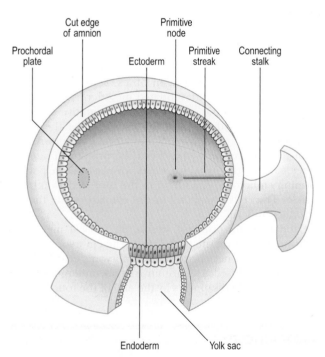

Fig. 5.2 Dorsal view of a 16-day embryo. (From Mitchell B, Sharma R. *Embryology: An Illustrated Colour Text.* 2nd ed. London: Elsevier; 2009. Fig. 1.7.)

the prechordal plate where the ectoderm and endoderm are fused. Prechordal mesoderm is formed from mesenchymal population of neural crest origin, rostral to the notochord. Mesenchymal cells from the primitive streak and notochordal process also migrate laterally and cranially, until they reach the margins of the embryonic disc and become continuous with the extraembryonic mesoderm covering the amnion and umbilical vesicle. Other mesenchymal cells also migrate cranially and around the prechordal plate where they form cardiogenic mesoderm.

By the middle of the third week, intraembryonic mesoderm separates the ectoderm and endoderm everywhere except at the oropharyngeal membrane, in the median plane cranial to the primitive node where the notochordal process is located, and at the cloacal membrane.

The primitive pit continues to develop and extend into the notochordal process, forming the notochordal canal. The floor of the notochord and the underlying embryonic endoderm fuse and gradually undergo apoptosis (Fig. 5.5A), resulting in the formation of confluent openings in the floor of the notochordal process. This brings the notochordal canal into communication with the umbilical vesicle and results in the loss of the floor of the notochordal canal. The notochordal process then becomes a flattened, grooved notochordal plate. Beginning at the cranial end, the notochordal plate cells proliferate and undergo infolding, which creates the notochord (Fig. 5.5B). The notochord further defines the primordial longitudinal axis of the embryo, gives some rigidity to the embryo, provides signals for development of axial musculoskeletal structures and the central nervous system, and contributes to the intervertebral discs. The developing notochord induces the overlying embryonic ectoderm to thicken and form the neural plate, the primordium of the central nervous system (CNS).

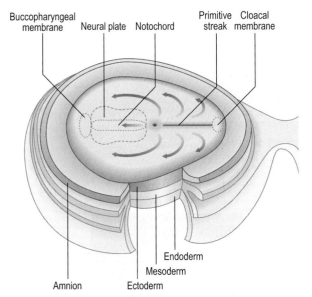

Fig. 5.3   Drawing of a transverse cut of the cranial half of the embryo to show migration of mesenchymal cells. (From Mitchell B, Sharma R. *Embryology: An Illustrated Colour Text.* 2nd ed. London: Elsevier; 2009. Fig. 1.8.)

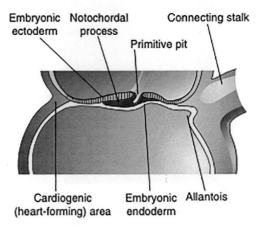

Fig. 5.4   Drawing of the median section of a 16-day embryo showing developing notochordal process. (Modified from Moore KL, Persaud TVN, & Torchia MG. *The Developing Human: Clinically Oriented Embryology.* 10th ed. Philadelphia: Elsevier; 2015. Fig. 4.8B.)

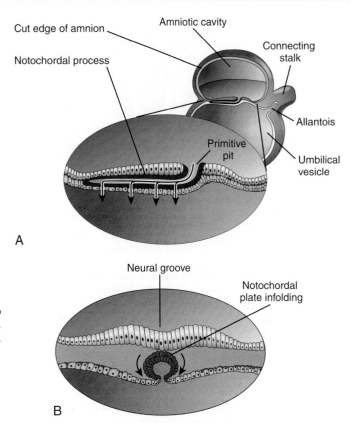

Fig. 5.5   (A) Drawing of the median section of an 18-day embryo showing apoptosis of floor of notochordal process. (B) Drawing of the transverse section of a slightly older embryo showing formation of the notochord and neural plate. (Modified from Moore KL, Persaud TVN, & Torchia MG. *The Developing Human: Clinically Oriented Embryology.* 10th ed. Philadelphia: Elsevier; 2015. Fig. 4.9.)

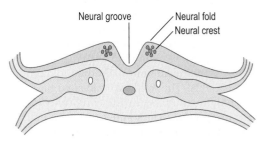

Fig. 5.6   Drawing of the transverse section of the embryo. (Modified from Mitchell B, Sharma R. *Embryology: An Illustrated Colour Text.* 2nd ed. London: Elsevier; 2009. Fig. 1.10A.)

NEURULATION

Neurulation is the process that forms the neural plate, neural folds, and then closure of the folds to form the neural tube. Neurulation is completed by the end of the fourth week, when closure of the caudal neuropore occurs.

The notochord induces the overlying embryonic ectoderm to form the neuroectoderm—an elongated plate of thickened epithelial cells that gives rise to the CNS, the brain, spinal cord and various other structures, including those of the eye. As the notochord elongates, the neural plate broadens and eventually extends cranially as far as the oropharyngeal membrane. Over time, the neural plate extends beyond the notochord.

Around day 18, the neural plate invaginates along its central axis to form a neural groove with bilateral neural folds (Fig. 5.6). The neural folds become particularly prominent at the cranial end of the embryo and are the first signs of brain development. By day 21, the neural folds have begun to fuse, converting the neural plate into the neural tube (Fig. 5.7), the primordium of the brain vesicles and spinal cord. The neural tube soon separates from the surface ectoderm, the latter of which differentiates into the epidermis. Neurulation is completed during the fourth week.

Selected neuroectodermal cells on the crest of the merging neural folds undergo epithelial-to-mesenchymal transition and migrate away. As the neural tube separates from the surface ectoderm, these neural crest cells form a flattened irregular mass, the neural crest, between the neural tube and the overlying surface ectoderm (Fig. 5.7). The neural

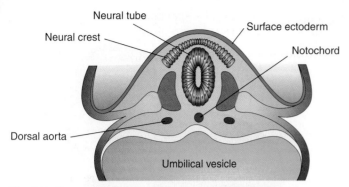

Fig. 5.7 Transverse section of the 22-day-old embryo showing neural tube and neural crest. (Modified from Moore KL, Persaud TVN, & Torchia MG. *The Developing Human: Clinically Oriented Embryology.* 10th ed. Philadelphia: Elsevier; 2015. Fig. 17.1F.)

crest soon separates into right and left parts that shift to the dorsolateral aspects of the neural tube. Neural crest cells differentiate and migrate widely. Neural crest cells give rise to the spinal ganglia (dorsal root ganglia) and ganglia of the autonomic nervous system. Ganglia of cranial nerves V, VII, IX and X are also partly derived from neural crest cells. In addition, neural crest cells form the neurolemma sheaths of peripheral nerves and contribute to the formation of the leptomeninges, the arachnoid mater and pia mater. Neural crest cells also contribute to the formation of pigment cells, the suprarenal medulla and many other tissues and organs.

SOMITES

In addition to forming the notochord, cells derived from the primitive node form the paraxial mesoderm. This cell population appears as a thick, longitudinal column of cells continuous with the intermediate mesoderm and with the extraembryonic mesoderm covering the umbilical vesicle and amnion. Toward the end of the third week, the paraxial mesoderm differentiates, condenses and in a craniocaudal sequence begins to divide into paired cuboidal bodies, the somites (Fig. 5.8A). The somites are located on each side of the developing neural tube. By the end of the fifth week, 42 to 44 pairs are present. The somites form distinctive surface elevations (Fig. 5.8B) on the embryo. Somites give rise to most of the axial skeleton and associated musculature, as well as to the adjacent dermis of the skin. The first pair of somites appears a short distance caudal to the site at which the otic placode forms. Motor axons from the developing spinal cord innervate muscle cells in the somites.

PRIMITIVE CIRCULATORY SYSTEM

At the end of the second week, embryonic nutrition is derived from maternal blood by diffusion through the extraembryonic coelom and umbilical vesicle. Shortly after, blood vessel formation begins in the extraembryonic mesoderm of the umbilical vesicle, connecting stalk and chorion, and then in the embryo. Early formation of the cardiovascular system is correlated with the urgent need for blood vessels to provide oxygen and nourishment to the embryo from the maternal circulation.

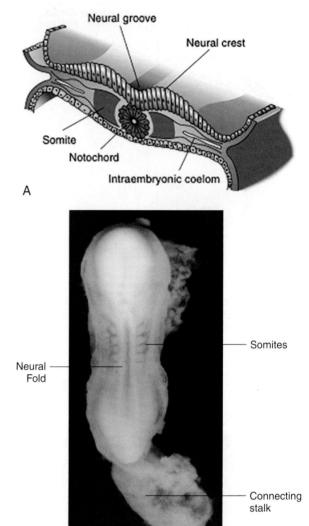

Fig. 5.8 (A) Transverse section of a 20-day-old embryo showing location of somite. (B) Dorsal view of an embryo (approximately 22 days) showing five pairs of somites. (Modified from Moore KL, Persaud TVN, & Torchia MG. *The Developing Human: Clinically Oriented Embryology.* 10th ed. Philadelphia: Elsevier; 2015. Figs 4.10, 5.6)

The formation of the embryonic vascular system involves vasculogenesis, the formation of new vascular channels by assembly of individual angioblasts (endothelial cell precursors) and angiogenesis, the formation of new vessels by budding from preexisting vessels. Blood vessel formation begins when mesenchymal cells differentiate into angioblasts which aggregate to form isolated angiogenic cell clusters, or blood islands. The angioblasts flatten to form endothelial cells that arrange themselves around the blood island cavities, forming the endothelium. Many of these cavities soon fuse to form networks of endothelial channels (vasculogenesis). Additional vessels sprout into adjacent areas (angiogenesis) and fuse with other vessels forming communicating channels. The mesenchymal cells surrounding the primordial endothelial blood vessels differentiate into the muscular and connective tissue elements of the vessels.

Haematogenesis occurs through specialised endothelial cells (hemangiogenic epithelium) of blood vessels as they grow on the umbilical vesicle and allantois and later in specialised sites along the dorsal aorta of the embryo. Progenitor blood cells also arise directly from hemangiopoietic stem cells. Blood formation begins in the embryo in the fifth week, first along the aorta and then in the liver, and later in the spleen, bone marrow and lymph nodes.

The heart and great vessels form from mesenchymal cells in the cardiogenic area. Paired, longitudinal endothelial-lined channels (endocardial heart tubes) develop during the third week and fuse to form a primordial heart tube, which joins with blood vessels in the embryo, connecting the stalk, chorion and umbilical vesicle to form a primordial cardiovascular system (Fig. 5.9B). By the end of the third week, blood is circulating, and the heart begins to beat on the 21st or 22nd day. The cardiovascular system is the first

organ system to reach a functional state. Motion of the primordial heart can be detected using ultrasonography during the fourth week.

CHORIONIC VILLI

Shortly after primary chorionic villi appear at the end of the second week, they begin to branch and become invested with mesenchymal cells. These secondary chorionic villi (Fig. 5.9A) cover the entire surface of the chorionic sac. Some of these mesenchymal cells soon differentiate into capillaries and blood cells, converting the secondary villi into tertiary villi (Fig. 5.9B). The capillaries in these chorionic

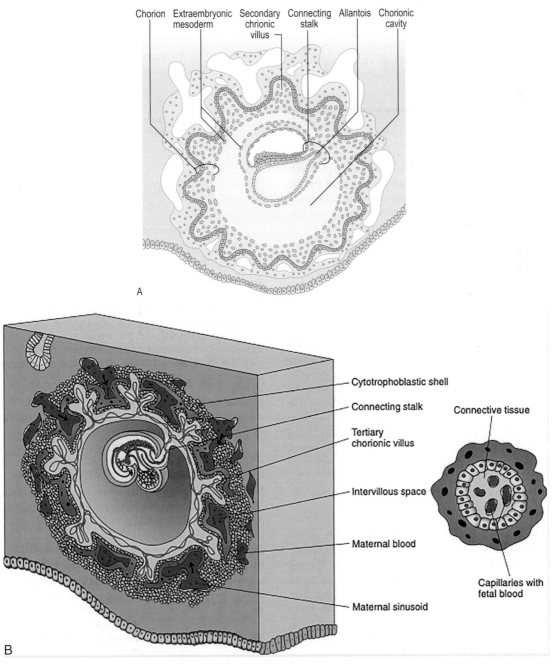

Fig. 5.9   (A) Drawing of a sagittal section of an embryo (16 days) showing secondary villi. (B) Drawing of a sagittal section of an embryo (21 days) tertiary villi. (Modified from Mitchell B, Sharma R. *Embryology: An Illustrated Colour Text.* 2nd ed. London: Elsevier; 2009. Fig. 2.2B.)

villi fuse to form arteriocapillary networks which connect with the embryonic heart through further vessel differentiation, including vessels in the stalk. By the end of the third week, embryonic blood begins to flow slowly through the capillaries in the chorionic villi. Oxygen and nutrients in the maternal plasma in the intervillous spaces diffuse through the walls of the villi and enter the embryo's blood. Carbon dioxide and waste products diffuse from blood in the fetal capillaries through the wall of the chorionic villi into the maternal blood.

Concurrently, cytotrophoblastic cells of the chorionic villi proliferate and extend through the syncytiotrophoblast to form an extravillous cytotrophoblastic shell which gradually surrounds the chorionic sac and attaches it to the endometrium. Villi that attach to the maternal tissues through the cytotrophoblastic shell are called stem or anchoring villi. The villi that grow from the sides of the stem villi are called branch villi, through which the main exchange of material between the blood of the mother and embryo takes place. The branch villi are bathed in continually changing maternal blood in the intervillous space.

FOLDING

Establishment of body form requires folding of the trilaminar embryonic disc into a somewhat cylinder-shaped embryo. Folding occurs in the median and horizontal planes and results from rapid growth of the embryo (Fig. 5.10A–C). Folding at the cranial and caudal ends and sides of the embryo occurs simultaneously, and it results in the cranial and caudal regions migrating ventrally, as the embryo elongates cranially and caudally (see Video 5.2).

CRANIAL FOLDING

At the beginning of the fourth week, the developing brain projects dorsally into the amniotic cavity. It grows cranially beyond the oropharyngeal membrane and overhangs the developing heart beginning the head folding. At the same time, the septum transversum, primordial heart, pericardial coelom and oropharyngeal membrane migrate onto the ventral surface of the embryo (Fig. 5.10A). During this folding, part of the endoderm of the umbilical vesicle is incorporated into the embryo as the foregut. After head folding, the septum transversum lies caudal to the heart, where it subsequently develops into the central tendon of the diaphragm.

CAUDAL FOLDING

This results primarily from growth of the distal part of the neural tube. The caudal eminence (tail region) projects over the cloacal membrane, the future site of the anus. During caudal folding (Fig. 5.10B), part of the endodermal germ layer is incorporated into the embryo as the hindgut. The terminal part of the hindgut soon dilates slightly to form the cloaca, the rudiment of the urinary bladder and rectum. The connecting stalk (primordium of the umbilical cord) is now attached to the ventral surface of the embryo, and the allantois, or the diverticulum of the umbilical vesicle, is partially incorporated into the embryo.

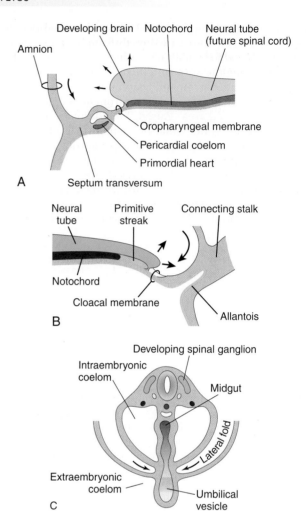

Fig. 5.10 (A) Drawing of a sagittal section of the cranial end of the embryo. The *arrows* indicates cranial folding and movement of the septum transversum, heart and other structures moving onto the ventral surface of the embryo. (B) Drawing of a sagittal section of the caudal end of the embryo. The *arrows* indicates caudal folding and movement of the cloacal membrane and primordial hindgut onto the ventral surface of the embryo. (C) Drawing of a transverse section of the embryo. *Arrows* indicate bilateral folding and initiation of the envelopment of a portion of the umbilical vesicle into the embryo. (Modified from Moore KL, Persaud TVN, & Torchia MG. *The Developing Human: Clinically Oriented Embryology*. 10th ed. Philadelphia: Elsevier; 2015. Figs 5.2, 5.4, 5.1C3.)

HORIZONTAL PLANE FOLDING

Lateral folding is produced by the rapidly growing spinal cord and somites. The primordia of the ventrolateral abdominal wall fold toward the median plane (Fig. 5.10C), rolling the edges of the embryonic disc ventrally and forming a roughly cylindrical embryo. As the abdominal wall forms, part of the endoderm germ layer is incorporated into the embryo as the midgut. Initially, there is a wide connection between the midgut and umbilical vesicle; however, after lateral folding, the connection is reduced, forming an omphaloenteric duct. The region of attachment of the amnion to the ventral surface of the embryo is also reduced to a relatively narrow umbilical region. As the umbilical cord forms from the connecting stalk, ventral fusion of the lateral folds reduces the region of communication between the intraembryonic and extraembryonic coelomic cavities to a narrow communication. As the amniotic cavity expands and obliterates most of the extraembryonic coelom, the amnion forms the epithelial covering of the umbilical cord.

Molecular Biology Considerations

- BMPs, FGFs, Shh, Tbx16, Tgifs and Wnts—gastrulation
- Wnt3a, Wnt5a and FGFs—germ cell layer fates
- TGF-β (nodal), veg T and Wnt—endoderm specification
- TGF-β superfamily, BMP4—mesoderm formation
- WNT, FGF, NOTCH, HOX, Tbx6—somite formation
- Wnt/β-catenin—neural crest development
- FOXD3, SNAIL2, SOX9, SOX10—differentiation and migration neural crest cells
- Delta-Notch signalling—craniocaudal sequencing of somite formation
- Fit1—anastomosis of primitive vessels

CLINICAL ISSUES

TERATOMA

Remnants of the primitive streak may persist and give rise to a sacrococcygeal teratoma, a type of germ cell tumour that may be benign or malignant. By definition, the tumours contain tissues derived from all three germ layers in varying stages of differentiation, as they arise from pluripotent cell lines. Sacrococcygeal teratomas are the most common congenital tumour in neonates and have an incidence of approximately 1 in 35,000 with a 4:1 preponderance in females. The teratomas are usually diagnosed on routine antenatal ultrasonography, with about 70% being benign. Usually, teratomas are promptly surgically excised, with the prognosis dependent on many factors. These presacral tumours may cause intestinal or urinary obstruction, and surgical excision of such masses can have long-term sequelae in terms of normal function of these systems.

SPONTANEOUS ABORTION

Spontaneous abortion (miscarriage) is pregnancy loss that occurs within the first 12 completed weeks of pregnancy and has a frequency of 25% to 30%. Approximately 80%

of spontaneous abortions of embryos occur during the first trimester. The true frequency of early spontaneous abortion is difficult to establish because it often occurs before a woman is aware that she is pregnant, but rates of 50% to 70% have been reported. A spontaneous abortion occurring several days after the first missed period is very likely to be mistaken for a delayed menstruation. More than half of all known spontaneous abortions result from chromosomal abnormalities of the embryo. The higher incidence of early spontaneous abortions in older women probably results from the increasing frequency of nondisjunction during oogenesis. Spontaneous abortions that result from failure of blastocysts to implant may result from a poorly developed endometrium and immune intolerance; however, in many cases, there are probably lethal chromosomal abnormalities in the embryo. There is a higher incidence of spontaneous abortion of fetuses with neural tube defects, cleft lip and cleft palate. After 10 gestational weeks, 25% to 40% of spontaneous abortions are related to fetal causes, 25% to 35% to placental causes and 5% to 10% to maternal causes, with the remainder unexplained.

CHORDOMAS

A chordoma is a rare malignancy that may form from vestigial remnants of the notochord. Approximately one-third of chordomas occur at the base of the cranium and extend to the nasopharynx. Chordomas grow slowly and may infiltrate adjacent bone and soft tissues.

Case Outcome

Measurement of serum β human chorionic gonadotropin (ß-hCG) showed a level of 12,200 mIU/mL. A transvaginal ultrasound was carried out, demonstrating an apparent abnormal gestational sac within the cervical canal. Based on the clinical work-up, JM was diagnosed with an incomplete spontaneous abortion.

Additional reflection: In what clinical situations would either expectant, medical or surgical treatment be recommended for an incomplete spontaneous abortion? What would you recommend as treatment, if any, for JM and why? What are the most common reasons for spontaneous abortion?

QUESTIONS

1. Which of the following is correct as it relates to gastrulation?
   a. The formation of the primitive groove is the first morphologic sign of gastrulation
   b. The primitive streak follows the formation of the primitive groove and is formed by hypoblast cells
   c. Some cells of the primitive streak leave its deep surface to form mesenchyme
   d. Cells from the hypoblast as well as from the primitive streak displace the hypoblast to form the ectoderm
   e. The primitive node is formed at the caudal end of the primitive streak.

2. During neurulation:
   a. the notochord forms the neural plate and neural folds
   b. the notochord induces the endoderm to form neuro-endoderm
   c. the neural folds first begin to fuse by day 28
   d. neural crest cells are formed by epithelial-to-mesenchymal transition of neuroectoderm
   e. neural crest cells form and remain adjacent to the neural tube

BIBLIOGRAPHY

Behera MA, Price TM. Abnormal (dysfunctional) uterine bleeding. Medscape. http://emedicine.medscape.com/article/257007. December 7, 2018.

Dupin E, Calloni GW, Coelho-Aguiar JM, Le Douarin NM. The issue of the multipotency of the neural crest cells. Dev Biol 2018; 444 Suppl 1:S47–59.

Vijayraghavan DS, Davidson L. Mechanics of neurulation: From classical to current perspectives on the physical mechanics that shape, fold, and form the neural tube. Birth Defects Res 2017;109(2):153–68.

Yoon HM, Byeon SJ, Hwang JY, et al. Sacrococcygeal teratomas in newborns: a comprehensive review for the radiologists. Acta Radiol 2018;59:236–46.

Placentation and Membranes | 6

Case Scenario

An anxious 34-year-old woman (TJ), 6-weeks pregnant, presents to the emergency department with vaginal bleeding that had begun 5 hours earlier. TJ described mild lower quadrant abdominal pain, but no other symptoms. Six months previously, she had had a spontaneous abortion at 8 weeks gestation. Otherwise, her past medical history was unremarkable. TJ was taking no medications, did not smoke and denied any alcohol or illicit drug use.

All vital signs were normal. Abdominal examination demonstrated no tenderness or distension, and normal bowel sounds. The uterus was not palpable. Pelvic examination demonstrated a closed cervical os; scant blood was noted in the vaginal vault with no active bleeding. The remainder of the physical examination was unremarkable.

Haematology and blood chemistry results were normal. Urinalysis revealed no white cells, a few red blood cells and a few bacteria (nitrite, ketones and glucose were all negative). Serum β human chorionic gonadotrophin (β-hCG) was 17,230 mIU/mL. An ultrasound examination using an endovaginal probe was conducted and demonstrated two fluid-filled structures in the uterus measuring 1.7 cm × 0.8 cm and 2.2 cm × 0.5 cm. The remainder of the ultrasound examination was normal.

Questions for reflection: Does a previous spontaneous abortion increase the risk for future spontaneous abortions? What is the significance of the red blood cells and bacteria in the urine sample and the β-hCG result? What is the significance of a closed cervix on pelvic examination? What could the two fluid-filled structures represent?

PLACENTATION AND MEMBRANES

The placenta, a fetomaternal organ, is comprised of a fetal part that develops from the chorionic sac and a maternal part derived from the decidua basalis (the part of the endometrium that is deep to the conceptus). Early development of the placenta is characterised by rapid proliferation of trophoblast and development of the chorionic sac and chorionic villi. By the end of the third week, the basic components necessary for physiological exchanges between the mother and embryo are established.

Chorionic villi cover the entire chorionic sac until the beginning of the eighth week (Fig. 5.8). As the chorionic sac grows, the villi associated with the decidua capsularis (decidua overlying the embryo) become compressed, necrotic and degenerate, producing the smooth chorion. The villi of the decidua basalis then rapidly proliferate, branch and enlarge, which forms the villous chorion (Fig. 5.9A). The placenta typically has a discoid shape. The fetal and maternal parts of the placenta are attached by the cytotrophoblastic shell, the external layer of trophoblastic cells on the maternal surface of the placenta. The chorionic villi are attached firmly to the decidua basalis through this shell. Endometrial arteries and veins pass freely through gaps in the cytotrophoblastic shell and enter the intervillous space (Fig. 6.3). As chorionic villi invade the decidua basalis, decidual tissue is eroded to enlarge the intervillous space. The placental septa, which project towards the chorionic plate, divide the fetal part of the placenta into cotyledons, each consisting of two or more stem villi and many branch villi. By the end of the fourth month, the decidua basalis is almost entirely replaced by cotyledons.

As the conceptus enlarges, the decidua capsularis bulges into the uterine cavity and becomes greatly attenuated. The decidua capularis eventually fuses with the decidua parietalis on the opposing uterine wall, obliterating the uterine cavity. By 22 to 24 weeks the decidua capsularis degenerates because of reduced vascularisation, allowing the smooth chorion to fuse with the decidua parietalis.

Initially, when trophoblastic cells invade the uterine spiral arteries, these cells create plugs within the arteries. The plugs allow only maternal plasma to enter the intervillous space. As a result, there is a net negative oxygen gradient created. Elevated oxygen levels during the early stages of development can be deleterious to the embryo. By 11 to 14 weeks, the plugs begin to break down, maternal whole blood begins to flow and oxygen concentrations increase.

The intervillous space (Fig. 6.3) of the placenta, which by 11 to 14 weeks contains maternal blood, results from the coalescence and enlargement of the lacunar networks. The intervillous space is partially divided into compartments by placental septa. Maternal blood enters the intervillous space from the spiral endometrial arteries in the decidua basalis. The intervillous space is drained by endometrial veins. The numerous branch villi are continuously bathed with maternal blood in the intervillous space. The branch chorionic villi provide a large surface area for exchange across the very thin placental membrane, consisting of extrafetal tissues, interposed between the fetal and maternal circulations. Until approximately 20 weeks, the placental membrane consists of four layers: syncytiotrophoblast, cytotrophoblast, connective tissue of the villi and endothelium of fetal capillaries. After the 20th week, the cytotrophoblastic cells disappear over large areas of the villi, leaving only thin patches of syncytiotrophoblast. As a result, the placental membrane then consists of three layers in most areas, and in some sites the placental membrane becomes markedly attenuated. At these sites, the syncytiotrophoblast comes into direct contact with the endothelium of the fetal capillaries to form a vasculosyncytial placental membrane.

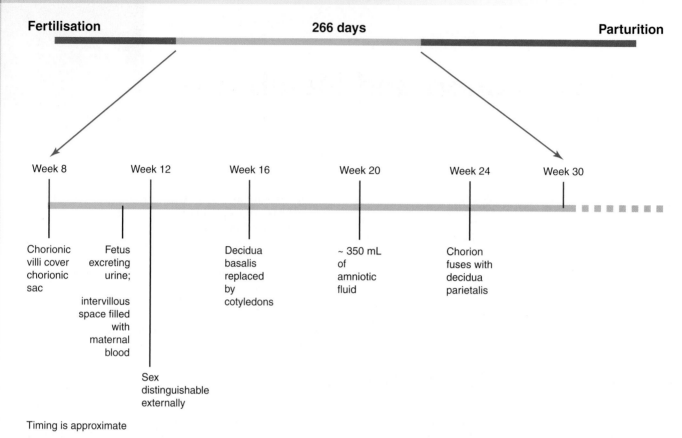

Fig. 6.1   Timeline of development related to placentation and formation of membranes.

PLACENTA AND IMMUNITY

The fetal parts of the placenta contain both paternal and maternal genes and therefore must be protected from the maternal immune system to prevent rejection. Although evidence continues to be discovered about the immune mechanisms necessary, there is some evidence to indicate:

- syncytiotrophoblast lacks major histocompatibility (MHC) antigens and thus does not evoke rejection responses
- local immunosuppressor molecules, PGE_2, TGF-β and interleukin 10, help to block activation of maternal T cells and natural killer (NK) cells
- activated maternal leukocytes are destroyed by apoptosis-inducing ligands present on the trophoblast
- complement regulatory proteins protect the placenta from complement-mediated destruction
- there is silencing of key maternal T cell-attracting inflammatory chemokine genes in decidual stromal cells.

FETAL AND MATERNAL PLACENTAL CIRCULATION

Deoxygenated blood from the fetus is carried to the placenta through the paired umbilical arteries (Fig. 6.3). The umbilical arteries divide into radially dispersed, branching chorionic arteries that enter the chorionic villi, forming an extensive arteriocapillary–venous network. This network brings the fetal blood extremely close to the maternal blood, separated only by the placental membrane. The reoxygenated blood in the capillaries passes into thin-walled veins that follow the chorionic arteries to the site of attachment of the umbilical cord. Here they converge to form the umbilical vein and carry oxygen-rich blood to the fetus.

The maternal blood in the intervillous space enters through 80 to 100 spiral endometrial arteries (Fig. 6.3) in the decidua basalis, which eject blood at a considerably higher pressure than that in the intervillous space. As a result, blood spurts towards the chorionic plate and then flows slowly over the branch villi, allowing exchange. The intervillous space of the mature placenta contains approximately 150 mL of blood, which is replenished three or four times per minute. The maternal blood eventually returns through the endometrial veins to the maternal circulation.

PLACENTAL FUNCTION AND TRANSPORTATION

The placenta has several main functions including metabolism, transportation of gases and nutrients, endocrine secretion, protection and excretion, all of which are essential for maintaining pregnancy and normal fetal development.

Particularly during early pregnancy, the placenta synthesises glycogen, cholesterol and fatty acids, which serve as sources of nutrients and energy for the fetus. These are also required for transport and endocrine secretion activities.

The placenta has a number of protective mechanisms, such as DNA methylation, which allow it to react to various environmental conditions (e.g., hypoxia) and exposures that may occur and minimise any impact on the fetus.

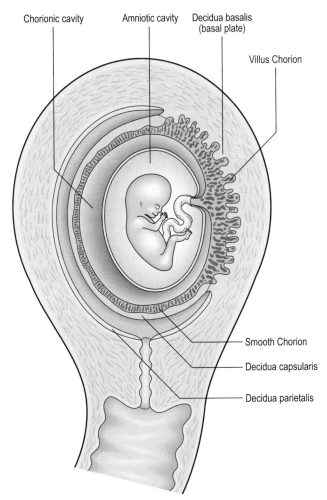

Chorionic cavity   Amniotic cavity   Decidua basalis (basal plate)

Villus Chorion

Smooth Chorion

Decidua capsularis

Decidua parietalis

Fig. 6.2 Drawing of a sagittal section of a uterus at 16 weeks showing the various membranes and placental structures. (Modified from Mitchell B, Sharma R. *Embryology: An Illustrated Colour Text.* 2nd ed. London: Elsevier; 2009. Fig. 2.1.)

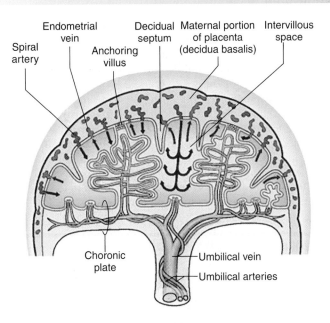

Endometrial vein   Decidual septum   Maternal portion of placenta (decidua basalis)   Intervillous space

Spiral artery   Anchoring villus

Choronic plate   Umbilical vein   Umbilical arteries

Fig. 6.3 Schematic drawing of a transverse section through a full-term placenta showing the relationship between the fetal and maternal parts of the placenta. (Modified from Mitchell B, Sharma R. *Embryology: An Illustrated Colour Text.* 2nd ed. London: Elsevier; 2009. Fig. 2.6A.)

There are only very few substances, endogenous or exogenous, that are unable to pass through the placental membrane; it acts as a true barrier only when a molecule is of a certain size, configuration and charge. Some substances present in the maternal circulation only pass through the placental membrane in quantities insufficient to affect the fetus. Most drugs and other substances in the maternal blood plasma pass through the placental membrane and enter the fetal blood plasma. Almost all materials are transported across this membrane by one of the following four main transport mechanisms:

• simple diffusion—passive transport characteristic of substances moving from areas of higher to lower concentration until equilibrium
• facilitated diffusion—transport through electrical gradients requiring a transporter but no energy
• active transport—passage of ions or molecules across a cell membrane against a concentration gradient and requires energy (e.g., ATP)
• pinocytosis—a form of endocytosis where the material is a small amount of extracellular fluid and usually reserved for large molecules

There are other ways that cells may transfer across the placental membrane. Erythrocytes (maternal or fetal) can enter the fetal or maternal circulation through small defects in the placental membrane. Maternal leukocytes may cross under their own power. Some bacteria and protozoa such as *Toxoplasma gondii* create placental lesions and then cross the membrane through the resulting defects.

Water and gases cross the placental membrane by simple diffusion. The quantity of oxygen reaching the fetus is primarily limited by blood flow (maternal or fetal) rather than oxygen diffusion. Glucose produced by both the mother and the placenta is quickly transferred by facilitated (active) diffusion mediated primarily by glucose transporter 1 (GLUT1). Amino acids are actively transported across the placental membrane; for most amino acids, the plasma concentrations in the fetus are higher than in the mother. Water-soluble vitamins cross the placental membrane more quickly than fat-soluble vitamins. Unconjugated steroid hormones cross the placental membrane quite freely. Protein hormones (e.g., insulin) reach the fetus in only very small amounts, except thyroxine and triiodothyronine which enter by slow transfer. Electrolytes are freely exchanged across the placental membrane in significant quantities, each type at its own rate. Transferrin crosses the placental membrane (placental receptors) and carries iron to the embryo/fetus. Urea and uric acid pass through the placental membrane by simple diffusion. Conjugated bilirubin is easily transported.

The immaturity of the fetal immune system means that only small quantities of antibodies are produced. However, some degree of passive immunity is provided by the transfer of maternal IgG gamma globulins by transcytosis, beginning at 16 weeks and peaking at 26 weeks.

The amount of drugs or metabolites crossing the placental membrane is controlled by the maternal blood concentration and the blood flow through the placenta because most such compounds cross by simple diffusion. Most drugs used for the management of labour readily cross the placental membrane. Viruses may pass through the placental membrane and cause fetal infection. Microorganisms such as *Treponema pallidum* and *T. gondii* also cross the placental membrane.

The placenta synthesises progesterone and oestrogens. The syncytiotrophoblast produces oestrogen and protein hormones including chorionic gonadotropin (hCG), chorionic somatomammotropin (hCS) and chorionic thyrotropin (hCT). hCG maintains the corpus luteum, hCS causes decreased maternal glucose utilisation and increased maternal free fatty acids whereas hCT appears to function similarly to thyroid-stimulating hormone.

AMNIOTIC CAVITY AND FLUID

The amniotic sac that surrounds the developing embryo and fetus contains amniotic fluid.

Because the amniotic sac enlarges faster than the chorionic sac, the amnion and smooth chorion fuse to form the amniochorionic membrane which, in turn, fuses with the decidua capsularis. It is the amniochorionic membrane that ruptures during labour. The amnion also forms the epithelial covering of the umbilical cord.

Initially, amniotic fluid is derived from maternal tissue and interstitial fluid by diffusion from the decidua parietalis; diffusion of fluid from blood in the intervillous space through the chorionic plate; tissue fluid from the fetus (before skin keratinisation); and fluid secreted by the fetal gastrointestinal and respiratory tracts, with the latter contributing approximately 350 mL/day. During the 11th week, the fetus begins to excrete urine into the amniotic cavity, with more than 0.5 L added daily, late in pregnancy. The total volume of amniotic fluid is approximately 30 mL at 10 weeks, 350 mL at 20 weeks and 700 to 1000 mL by 37 weeks.

The exchange of water content in amniotic fluid occurs continuously through the amniochorionic membrane into the maternal tissue fluid and then enters through uterine capillaries. Such an exchange also happens via fetal blood, through the umbilical cord and chorionic plate on the fetal surface of the placenta. Amniotic fluid is also swallowed and absorbed by the fetal digestive tracts, passing into the fetal bloodstream, with the waste products crossing the placental membrane into the maternal blood. Any excess water in the fetal blood is excreted by the fetal kidneys and returned to the amniotic sac through urination.

UMBILICAL CORD

Early in development the bilaminar embryo is surrounded by extraembryonic mesoderm, formed by the endodermal cells of the umbilical vesicle. At approximately 10 days, apoptosis occurs in the extraembryonic mesoderm, causing extraembryonic coelomic spaces to appear, which soon coalesce resulting in the bilaminar embryo being suspended within what will become the chorionic cavity. The embryo remains attached to the developing placenta by the connecting stalk. As the embryo develops, the amniotic sac enlarges and envelopes the connecting stalk and a portion of the umbilical vesicle, forming the umbilical cord. In addition, blood vessels, initially two veins and two arteries, are integrated into the umbilical cord through the processes of angiogenesis and vasculogenesis. By the end of the fifth week, the umbilical cord has blood flowing in these vessels. The right umbilical vein becomes obliterated by the sixth week, leaving a single vein, two arteries and the remnant of the umbilical vesicle, the allantois. The two arteries typically form a helical structure around the vein. Close to the placenta, there is also an anastomosis between the two arteries; it is thought that this acts as a pressure equaliser. The structure of the umbilical cord and patency of the blood vessels are supported by special connective tissue (Wharton's jelly). At term, the cord is typically 50 to 60 cm long (range of 30–100 cm), with a diameter of approximately 8 mm. In most cases, the umbilical cord connects to the centre of the placenta, but less commonly it may also connect closer to the margin.

Molecular Biology Considerations

- HLX, MSX2 and DLX3—expressed in the trophoblast induce trophoblastic invasion and regulate placental development
- MAP2K1, MAP2K2 and Gcm1—in trophoblast stem cells regulate the branching process of the stem villi
- EGF, TGF-α, amphiregulin, VEGF—stimulation of cytotrophoblast cell production
- TGF-β—binding leucine-rich proteoglycan decorin (DCN) reduces cytotrophoblast migration and invasiveness
- Human placental methylome—selectively regulates maternal and fetal exchanges; also controls fetal growth and development

---

CLINICAL ISSUES

HYPERTENSIVE DISORDERS OF PREGNANCY

PREECLAMPSIA AND ECLAMPSIA

Development of new hypertension ($\geq$140 mmHg systolic or $\geq$90 mmHg diastolic) after the 20th week of gestation in an otherwise normotensive woman is considered preeclampsia. It usually includes proteinuria. With increasing severity, it may also include thrombocytopenia, reduced liver or kidney function, pulmonary oedema or cerebral and/or visual symptoms. The origin of preeclampsia appears to be multifactorial; the primary pathology being a hypoinvasive placenta and compromised uterine angiogenesis leading to reduced placental perfusion and production of toxins that attack the maternal vasculature. The renal angiotensin system has also been implicated. Preeclampsia is a leading cause of maternal morbidity and may lead to fetal malnutrition, fetal growth restriction, miscarriage or fetal death. Eclampsia is diagnosed when seizures occur, without previous history, in a woman with preeclampsia. Eclampsia is a leading cause of maternal mortality.

GESTATIONAL HYPERTENSION

Gestational hypertension is defined as the development of hypertension ($\geq$140 mmHg systolic or $\geq$90 mmHg diastolic), without proteinuria, after the 20th week of gestation.

HELLP SYNDROME

HELLP syndrome is considered a variant of preeclampsia, where *h*aemolysis, *e*levated *l*iver transaminases and *low p*latelets occur without or without hypertension or proteinuria.

SUBCHORIONIC HAEMATOMA

Bleeding between the chorion and the uterus may occur, resulting in the development of a haematoma. It is a common cause of vaginal bleeding during the first 20 weeks of pregnancy. The haematoma can be seen during an ultrasound examination and is the most common abnormality seen in women with otherwise healthy pregnancies. Often, no symptoms present and the haematoma is detected during routine ultrasound examination. In most patients, any associated bleeding is self-limiting. Such bleeding occurring within the first 2 weeks of pregnancy is called an implantation bleed. Subchorionic haematomas can increase the risk of preterm labour or placental abruption.

PLACENTAL IMPLANTATION DEFECTS

PLACENTA PREVIA

In about 0.4% of pregnancies, the blastocyst implants at or near the internal os of the uterus, rather than at a location in the superior portion of the uterine cavity. In these cases, bright red but painless bleeding after 20 weeks of pregnancy is the common presenting symptom. Modified (reduced) physical activity is the initial treatment when symptoms occur before 36 weeks, after which time caesarean delivery is required. Caesarean delivery may also be necessary at earlier stages if the bleeding does not cease or if the health of the mother or fetus is threatened.

PLACENTA ACCRETA, INCRETA OR PERCRETA

When the chorionic villi penetrate beyond the normal decidual layer of the endometrium to the myometrium, the placenta is called placenta accreta (incidence 0.2%). In rarer cases, chorionic villi penetrate the full thickness of the myometrium (placenta increta) or to or through the serosa (placenta percreta). For delivery, a planned preterm caesarean hysterectomy is the recommended approach leaving the placenta in place to prevent massive bleeding. In exceptional circumstances, alternative approaches (e.g., medical therapy with high dose methotrexate) may preserve reproductive function but this also carries additional risk.

ISSUES OF THE UMBILICAL CORD

An umbilical cord that is too short has been associated with early placental separation, growth restriction and a number of fetal anomalies. An excessively long cord can become entangled, prolapse at parturition or loop around the fetal neck. In about 1% of pregnancies, the cord has only a single artery; 20% of these fetuses have a cardiovascular defect. Euploidy, growth restriction and renal anomalies are also associated with some cases of single artery cords. In some pregnancies, the umbilical cord is not connected directly to the placenta but rather enters the chorioamniotic membrane (velamentous insertion) with the umbilical vessels traversing between the amnion and chorion, and then connecting to the placenta. The vessels are not protected by Wharton's jelly and have an increased incidence of rupture, especially if the vessels are near the cervix (vasa previa). In these cases, a planned early caesarean delivery is recommended.

FETAL ERYTHROBLASTOSIS

Depending on the genetic makeup of the parents, a fetus may have Rh-positive blood type, while the mother is Rh negative. When small amounts of fetal blood enter the maternal circulation through microscopic breaks in the placental membrane, the fetal blood cells will stimulate the maternal immune system to produce anti-Rh antibodies. The antibodies can pass back through the placental membrane to the fetal blood, resulting in haemolysis of the fetal Rh-positive blood cells. Haemolysis (fetal erythroblastosis) leads to anaemia and jaundice. Severely affected fetuses may require early delivery or transfusions before and/or following birth. In pregnancies at risk, fetal erythroblastosis can be prevented by giving Rho(D) immunoglobulin to the mother. Fetal erythroblastosis may also result from fetomaternal incompatibilities of other blood antigen systems including Kell, Duffy, Xg and Cc; ABO blood type incompatibility does not cause fetal erythroblastosis.

OLIGOHYDRAMNIOS AND POLYHYDRAMNIOS

A reduced volume of amniotic fluid for a given gestational age (oligohydramnios) can result from placental insufficiency (diminished blood flow) or preterm rupture of the amniochorionic membrane. Obstructive uropathy or fetal renal agenesis will result in reduced or no urine input, respectively, to amniotic fluid and result in oligohydramnios. Compression of the fetus by the uterine wall because of reduced amniotic fluid can result in pulmonary hypoplasia and/or facial and limb defects, and compression of the umbilical cord. More severe consequences (lethal lung hyperplasia, eye malformation, heart defects) can be seen in fetuses with Potter sequence resulting from oligohydramnios.

Larger than normal volumes of amniotic fluid for a given gestational age (polyhydramnios; 1% of pregnancies) are caused by factors related to the fetus (e.g., oesophageal atresia, neurological defects), mother (diabetes) or be idiopathic. Complications of polyhydramnios include premature rupture of the membranes, preterm contractions, umbilical cord prolapse and increased risk of fetal death.

MULTIPLE GESTATION

The fertilisation of two oocytes leads to dizygotic (DZ) twins, which may be the same or different sexes. The incidence of DZ twins is quite variable (1:20–1:500) depending on race. DZ twins always have separate amnions and chorions although the latter may also be fused if they implant adjacent to each other, in which case the placentas may also be fused. Minor anastomoses between placental vessels may occur, resulting in erythrocyte mosaicism.

If a single oocyte occurs follow by division of the early embryo, monozygotic (MZ) twins develop; they have the same sex and are genetically identical, although because of other factors (e.g., unequal X-chromosome inactivation) they may be discordant for genetic disease or birth defects. If separation occurs at the blastomere stage, the MZ twins will have two amnions and chorions; two placentas also develop but may be fused if implantation is adjacent. More commonly, separation occurs at the blastocyst stage resulting in each embryos having an amniotic sac but a common chorionic sac (monochorionic–diamniotic) and a shared placenta. Twin transfusion syndrome can occur in monochorionic–diamniotic MZ twins when arterial blood is shunted from one twin to the other through unidirectional umbilical–placental arteriovenous anastomoses. The recipient will have polycythaemia and increased size while the donor will be anaemic and small; depending on the severity, either one twin or both could die. Fetoscopic laser coagulation of placental vascular anastomoses is the established method of management of twin transfusion syndrome. Rarely, separation of the embryo occurring at the later embryonic disc (week 2) results in monochorionic–monoamniotic twins; fetal mortality resulting from cord entanglement is significant. Very rarely, if the division of the embryonic disc is incomplete, various types of conjoined MZ twins may occur.

OTHER

PLACENTAL ABRUPTION

Partial or complete separation of the placenta (placental abruption; chronic or acute; 1% incidence) can result from abdominal trauma, polyhydramnios or premature rupture of the membranes. Other risk factors include maternal cocaine use, hypertension or intraamniotic infection. Placental abruption can result in severe maternal haemorrhage, shock and disseminated intravascular coagulopathy. If placental abruption is chronic, fetal distress may occur. Treatment of placental abruption ranges from modified maternal activity to vaginal delivery to emergency caesarean delivery and aggressive resuscitation, depending on the circumstances.

Case Outcome

Further information from the ultrasound examination included that one fluid-filled structure (1.7 cm × 0.8 cm) contained a fetal pole and fetal heart motion. It demonstrated a double decidual sign. The second sac contained a hyperechoic area resembling a fetal pole but without heart motion. The sonographer described one live intrauterine pregnancy and a subchorionic haemorrhage. One day later, a repeat ultrasound was performed that revealed that the subchorionic haemorrhage had decreased in size. TJ had no further vaginal bleeding in hospital and was discharged. Her pregnancy continued to full term with the delivery of a healthy boy.

Additional reflections: What is the aetiology and significance of a double decidual sign? Does the measured size of the conceptus match the date of pregnancy and β-hCG? What treatment is required for a subchorionic haemorrhage and what, if any are the long-term risks to the mother or the fetus? What is the risk to the embryo, at this age, from b-mode diagnostic ultrasound? What about the risks from Doppler ultrasound?

QUESTIONS

1. In dizygotic twins, which of the following is correct?
   a. They result from division of the embryoblast into two embryos
   b. They result from fertilisation of two ova by two sperms
   c. They usual begin to separate during the blastocyst stage
   d. These twins are usually identical
   e. Only one chorionic sac will be found

2. Which of the following statements related to the placenta is true?
   a. The intervillous space contains fetal and maternal blood
   b. As the embryo enlarges, the decidua parietalis is replaced by cotyledons
   c. Initially there is a net negative oxygen gradient because of spiral artery plugs
   d. Until 20 weeks, the placenta membrane consists of three layers
   e. Throughout pregnancy, chorionic villi cover the entire chorionic sac

3. Which of the following statements related to placental function and transportation is true?
   a. Almost all substances, endogenous or exogenous, are able to cross the placenta
   b. The placenta cannot synthesise glycogen and is therefore dependent on uterine glands for glycogen
   c. Oxygenation across the placenta is limited by diffusion rather than blood flow
   d. The placenta synthesises progesterone but not oestrogen, and is therefore reliant on the ovaries for oestrogen
   e. Glucose produced by the placenta is transported by simple diffusion

4. Which of the following statements is correct?
   a. Preeclampsia usually does not include proteinuria but may include reduced liver function
   b. Placenta previa occurs with implantation at or near the external uterine os
   c. Fetal erythroblastosis results from either Rh or ABO blood type incompatibility
   d. The main concern with a velamentous insertion of the umbilical cord is that the vessels are more prone to rupture
   e. Twin transfusion syndrome occurs more commonly in dizygotic twins with fused placentas than in monozygotic twins

BIBLIOGRAPHY

Berceanu C, Mehedinţu C, Berceanu S, et al. Morphological and ultrasound findings in multiple pregnancy placentation. Rom J Morphol Embryol 2018;59:435–53.

Nassar GN, Wehbe C. Erythroblastosis Fetalis. StatPearls [Internet]. Treasure Island (FL): StatPearls Publishing; 2019.

Vintzileos AM, Ananth CV, Smulian JC. Using ultrasound in the clinical management of placental implantation abnormalities. Am J Obstet Gynecol 2015;213(4 Suppl):S70–7.

Wiedaseck S, Monchek. Placental and cord insertion pathologies: screening, diagnosis, and management. J Midwifery Womens Health 2014;59:328–35.

Fetal and Neonatal Period

7

Case Scenario

A woman (gravida 2, para 1) presents to the local hospital in the early stages of full-term labour with the fetal membranes having ruptured 1 hour ago. The last fetal ultrasound examination was performed at 20 weeks gestation, demonstrating a normal female fetus; measurement of both abdominal circumference and biparietal diameters placed the fetus at the 40% percentile for each. Both parents were small for gestational age when born. Since 20 weeks gestation, and up to 1 week ago, the mother had travelled from her home in North America and had been living in rural Bangladesh, caring for an ill parent. She had received no further prenatal care. The mother had no significant past medical or obstetric history and did not smoke or use alcohol. Vaginal delivery of a female infant occurred without complication with Apgar scores of 8/9 (1/5 minutes). The infant's birth weight and abdominal circumference were all less than the 5th percentile whereas biparietal diameter and body length were within normal limits; her Ballard score is 37.

Questions for reflection. Would this neonate be considered constitutionally small for gestational age? What factors could have altered the normal growth during fetal development? In this case, with a normal ultrasound at 20 weeks, what factors, if any might be more likely? What implications does an asymmetric growth pattern carry? What information is provided by the Ballard score and how might it impact your diagnosis? What information in the mother's history might be important?

ASSESSMENT OF THE EMBRYO AND FETUS

In many countries, routine ultrasonography is offered to women at approximately 10 to 13 weeks gestation to determine gestation age, measure nuchal translucency (screening component for trisomy 21), and to detect multiple pregnancies and determine membrane characteristics. Scanning in the second trimester allows for detection of fetal anomalies such as neural tube defects, diaphragmatic hernia, cardiac anomalies, renal agenesis and cleft lip. When there is concern about the velocity of fetal growth or a more accurate determination of expected delivery date is required, ultrasonography can allow measurement of biparietal diameter, abdominal circumference, femur length or head circumference (most often used for determining gestation age). Ultrasound is the main diagnostic imaging modality for the evaluation of the embryo and fetus. Amniotic fluid volume measurements can be also be made, as can an assessment of fetal movements and placental appearance. Other ultrasound techniques such as Doppler ultrasound can be used to determine, for instance, blood flow across a heart valve or in the umbilical cord. Lastly, biopsy of fetal tissues or amniocentesis can be achieved, when necessary, using ultrasound guidance.

The use of magnetic resonance imaging (MRI) of the fetus has increased in the last decade as techniques have improved. MRI has been demonstrated to be safe for the fetus and provides greatly enhanced soft tissue resolution with a much larger field of view. It is most commonly used after approximately 17 weeks gestation as an adjunct to ultrasound for further analysis or clarification of diagnosed or suspected fetal anomalies.

In some circumstances, obtaining embryo or fetal cells is required to further evaluate for the presence of genetic disorders. In amniocentesis, a needle is passed, using ultrasound guidance, through the mother's abdominal and uterine walls, to pierce the amniotic sac and remove a small amount of fluid containing sloughed fetal cells. Amniocentesis is performed after sufficient fluid exists (≥ 15 weeks). The procedure carries a very small risk to the fetus (pregnancy loss of 0.5%–1.0%). Most commonly, amniocentesis is performed when the following conditions exist: advanced maternal age, parent(s) with chromosomal abnormality or history of previous pregnancies with neural tube or genetic defects.

Chorionic villus sampling (CVS) is another method to obtain fetal cells. During CVS, trophoblastic tissue is biopsied under ultrasound guidance, by inserting a needle or catheter into the uterine cavity (either transabdominal or transcervical, respectively). CVS can be performed earlier (at 10–12 weeks) than amniocentesis with similar low risk.

If assisted reproductive technology is used to facilitate conception, one of more blastomeres can be removed for study.

Cells obtained during any of these methods can be cultured and examined using chromosomal microarray analysis for detecting chromosomal abnormalities. Fetal sex determination is also of importance in diagnosing sex-linked hereditary diseases. Fluorescence in situ hybridisation (FISH) can be used to detect microdeletions or duplications and subtelomeric rearrangements. Inborn errors of metabolism and enzyme deficiencies can be detected by incubating cells and measuring specific enzyme activity.

In the fetus, α-fetoprotein (AFP) is synthesised primarily by the fetal liver and umbilical vesicle, and it the most abundant serum protein, with levels peaking at 12 weeks gestation. Maternal plasma levels of AFP peak shortly after the fetal levels. Amniotic AFP and maternal plasma AFP are

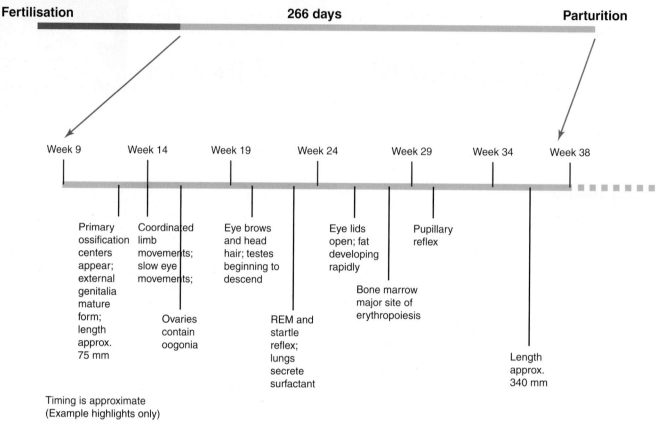

Fertilisation   **266 days**   **Parturition**

Week 9   Week 14   Week 19   Week 24   Week 29   Week 34   Week 38

Primary   Coordinated
ossification   limb
centers   movements;
appear;   slow eye
external   movements;
genitalia
mature   Ovaries
form;   contain
length   oogonia
approx.
75 mm

Eye brows
and head
hair; testes
beginning to
descend

REM and
startle
reflex;
lungs
secrete
surfactant

Eye lids
open; fat
developing
rapidly

Bone marrow
major site of
erythropoiesis

Pupillary
reflex

Length
approx.
340 mm

Timing is approximate
(Example highlights only)

Fig. 7.1   Timeline of development related to the fetal and neonatal period.

higher in fetuses with severe central nervous system and abdominal wall defects. Maternal AFP measurement is also helpful as a component of screening tests for fetal trisomy 21, trisomy 18 and other chromosome defects.

Fetal cells and cell-free fetal DNA and RNA can be found in maternal blood; as a result, DNA-based prenatal sequencing using chromosomal microarray analysis and whole-exome sequencing provide further means of screening for genetic abnormalities.

FETAL PERIOD

By definition, the fetal period begins at the start of gestational week 9. Although the majority of organ systems have completed their early development by the end of the embryonic period (end of week 8), maturation of the various systems continues. For example:

- Weeks 9–12: fetal urine begins to form, bipotential external genitalia have established the mature differentiated form, erythropoiesis expands in location from the liver to include the spleen
- Weeks 14–16: rapid growth, coordinated limb and slow-eye movements, scalp hair patterning completed
- Weeks 16–20: external ears are found at their final position, head hair and eyebrow are visible, brown fat forms
- Weeks 21–25: rapid eye movements, blink-startle response, pulmonary surfactant is being produced

- Weeks 26–29: breathing movements, eyelids open, erythropoiesis moves primarily to the bone marrow
- Weeks 30–34: pupillary reflex, increasing percent of body fat
- Weeks 35–38: fat represents approximately 15% body weight, testes located in scrotum.

PARTURITION

The term parturition (childbirth; labour and delivery) describes the process of expulsion of the fetus, placenta and fetal membranes from the mother. Labour is typically divided into three stages: cervical dilation (early and active labour), expulsion and the placental stage. The term 'delivery' denotes the second and third stages of labour.

The factors that trigger labour are not completely understood; however, several hormones, including relaxin (produced by the corpus luteum and placenta), are related to the initiation of contractions. The fetal hypothalamus secretes corticotropin-releasing hormone. This hormone stimulates the anterior hypophysis (pituitary) to produce adrenocorticotropin causing the secretion of cortisol from the suprarenal (adrenal) cortex. Cortisol is involved in the synthesis of oestrogens that are formed by the ovaries, placenta, testes and, possibly, adrenal cortex. Increasing oestrogens (decreased relative to progesterone concentration) impact myometrial contractile activity and stimulate the release of oxytocin and prostaglandins. Peristaltic contractions of uterine smooth muscle are elicited by oxytocin, a hormone released by the neurohypophysis of the pituitary gland. This hormone is administered clinically when it is necessary to induce labour. Oxytocin also stimulates release of prostaglandins (promoters of uterine contractions) from the decidua, increasing myometrial contractility by sensitising the myometrial cells to oxytocin.

Cellular changes must also occur in the uterus, including the development of intermyometrial cell gap junctions to coordinate and transmit contractile signals, changes in nitric oxide, calcium and blood flow, as well as collagen breakdown in the cervix.

STAGES OF LABOUR

CERVICAL DILATION

Regular mild uterine contractions begin that, over time, result in the thinning and initial dilation of the cervical os to approximately 6 cm. This early process may require days to hours and is shorter for subsequent pregnancies. Contractions then become more intense and frequent as the cervical canal dilates from about 6 cm to 10 cm, at which point it is fully dilated; this portion of stage one (active labour) may last 4 to 8 hours.

EXPULSION

During the second stage of labour, lasting a few minutes to hours, the fetus descends through the cervix and vagina and exits the mother.

PLACENTAL STAGE

The expulsion of the placenta and membranes requires approximately 5 to 30 minutes during which time mild contractions will continue to be felt. Retraction of the uterus reduces the area of placental attachment and a haematoma forms deep to the placenta, which separates the placenta from the uterine wall (spongy layer of the decidua basalis.)

After delivery, myometrial contraction occurs to constrict the uterine spiral arteries and prevent excessive uterine bleeding.

FETAL TO NEONATAL TRANSITION

The transition from in utero to life after birth occurs rapidly, involves several systems and results in significant physiological changes. These include respiratory and cardiovascular, as well as immunological and thermoregulatory changes.

Approximately 90% of infants are born without any problem adapting to extrauterine conditions, about 10% require some minor assistance to begin breathing, whereas 1% require extensive resuscitation. In utero, discontinuous fetal breathing movements (FBMs) contribute to the normal development of the lungs and mimic the activity of breathing. The exact mechanisms that initiate breathing at birth are not yet known, but a number of factors are believed to contribute, including physical stimuli (e.g., handling, mechanical compression of the chest during vaginal delivery, temperature changes), and CO_2 and $PcCO_2$ chemoreceptors (e.g., cord clamping). Clearance of fluid from the lungs occurs quickly. It is likely a result of inspiration-phase reduction of pressure in the intrapleural spaces and perialveolar interstitial spaces, causing fluid to move across the alveolar epithelium into the interstitium and then into the lymphatic system. The fluid is replaced by air and the functional residual capacity is maintained by both the action of surfactant and early breathing patterns such as breath holding, crying and expiratory braking.

Similar to the respiratory system, functional changes also occur in the cardiovascular system during fetal to neonatal transition. Breathing results in a series of circulatory changes. These include the reversal of blood flow in the foramen ovale and the ductus arteriosus (Fig. 8.12) and early functional closure of both shunts (with anatomical closure requiring many more days to weeks). Clamping of the umbilical cord triggers an increase in peripheral vascular resistance and increased blood pressure. The umbilical vessels also undergo quick functional closure. Deoxygenated blood then enters the right atrium through the inferior and superior vena cavae, passes from the right atrium into the right ventricle and continues via the pulmonary trunk for oxygenation in the lungs. The oxygenated blood is transported to the left atrium by the pulmonary veins, then to the left ventricle, and eventually enters the systemic circulation.

Recently, many guidelines have recommended delayed clamping (at least 30–60 seconds following birth) of the umbilical cord because this allows for approximately 75 to 100 mL of fetal blood to transfer from the placenta, increasing the neonatal haemoglobin levels and iron stores. In addition, immunoglobulin and stem-cell transfer are enhanced. With delayed clamping there is a slightly higher incidence of neonatal jaundice requiring phototherapy, but there is no indication of increasing the risk of maternal haemorrhage.

From a behavioural perspective, during the first hour of life the neonate shows strong sucking ability and is alert and active. A few hours later, the neonate tends to sleep for minutes to hours and may be difficult to rouse. Another active period follows again at 4 to 6 hours after birth.

Other transitions at birth include the loss of glucose supply from the mother's circulation. As a result, neonatal blood glucose levels will be lowest within the first 60 minutes and then stabilise some hours later with breast feeding combined with the utilisation of stored glycogen and fat.

Neonates have poorly developed thermoregulatory capacity because their ability to shiver is reduced. As a result, direct skin-to-skin physical contact with the mother is encouraged, as are warming blankets on the back and the use of head covering. Full-term neonates also have high levels of brown fat, containing high numbers of mitochondria, which can generate heat through fat metabolism.

Molecular Biology Considerations

- Activation of TLR9 within the placental membrane—release of proinflammatory mediators and lead to induction of labour
- 3,5-cAMP intracellular signalling, through PKA—inhibits myometrial cell contractility and suppresses uterine activity
- EGF, TGF and endothelin-1—act as inflammatory initiators for the chorioamniotic membrane
- Placental IGF1/2—fetal growth through endo- and autocrine stimulation

CLINICAL ISSUES

BIRTH WEIGHT AND INTRAUTERINE GROWTH

LOW BIRTH WEIGHT

The most common reason for neonatal death, after congenital anomalies, is low birth weight or short gestation (preterm delivery ≤37 weeks gestation). Low birth weight (LBW) is defined as a weight of less than 2500 g in a newborn; very low birth weight (VLBW) being <1500 g and extremely low birth weight (ELBW) at <1000 g. Newborns are considered small for gestational age (SGA) if their weight is less than the 10th weight percentile for their gestational age without specific consideration to intrauterine growth. Most of these SGA infants are simply constitutionally small with their weight dependent on race, genetics, sex or ethnicity, and at little or no risk; most catch up to their expected size by 2 years of age. SGA is not synonymous with LBW, VLBW or ELBW. For example, an infant born at 33 weeks weighing 1700 g would not be considered SGA (10th percentile of weight at 33 weeks = 1530 g) but would be considered LBW.

INTRAUTERINE GROWTH RESTRICTION

Restriction of fetal growth during in utero development can arise from fetal (e.g. chromosomal), maternal (e.g., nutrition, anaemia, gestational diabetes), placental (e.g., multiple gestations) or environmental (e.g., alcohol use, medications) factors, and it remains one of the leading causes of morbidity and mortality in the fetus and neonate. Intrauterine growth restriction (IUGR) can be asymmetric (~75% of cases) where, for instance, the reduction in growth occurs late in pregnancy and then mainly impacts weight gain rather than head or long bone growth. If the impacts occur early in pregnancy, a symmetrical pattern of IUGR will be established with all biometric indices impacted (e.g., femur length, head circumference)—these infants typically have higher morbidity rates. Serial examination by ultrasound measuring a variety of biometric indices is the best means of establishing and monitoring growth changes once clinical suspicion of IUGR is present. Complications of IUGR include higher risk of stillbirth, premature delivery and consequent perinatal events such as seizures, hypoglycaemia, thermoregulation issues, abnormal immunity and retinopathy. Beyond the immediate postpartum period, infants with a history of IUGR have an increased risk of cognitive and neurological issues. There is no specific treatment for IUGR beyond those that can be controlled and counselled for such as maternal alcohol consumption, smoking and nutritional supplementation.

LARGE FOR GESTATIONAL AGE

Newborns are considered large for gestational age (LGA) if their weight is greater than the 90th weight percentile for their gestational age. Some of these infants are simply constitutionally large with their weight dependent on race, genetics, sex or ethnicity. However, the most common cause for LGA infants is maternal gestational diabetes. Other factors may include maternal obesity, excessive pregnancy weight gain and rare fetal genetic anomalies. High levels of glucose reaching the fetus result in increased release of fetal insulin, which acts as a growth accelerant. Consequences of LGA include difficult delivery, birth trauma, neonatal hypoglycaemia (because of high fetal insulin levels without the maternal supply of glucose) and polycythaemia.

STILLBIRTH

The most common definition for stillbirth is fetal death at greater than 20 weeks gestation. Stillbirth may result from maternal (e.g., uncontrolled diabetes, preeclampsia), fetal (chromosomal defects, major malformations), placental (placental abruption) or environmental (maternal alcohol consumption) factors. Often, a specific cause will not be found, in spite of testing. Uterine evacuation may occur naturally or may have to be induced. Fragments of placenta may be retained and, if so, will require surgical removal by curettage. If the fetus dies and remains in the uterus for a number of weeks, potentially fatal maternal disseminated intravascular coagulation (DIC) may occur.

PRETERM LABOUR

Labour occurring between 20 and 37 weeks increases the risk to the fetus, and occurs in approximately 10% of pregnancies. There are a number of possible causes of preterm labour including premature rupture of the chorioamniotic membrane, preeclampsia, IUGR and placenta previa. In addition, there may be alterations in the control systems that allow the uterus to remain quiescent during pregnancy including increased concentrations of prostaglandins because of deficiency of its degradation enzyme, infection of the uterus or chorioamnion that leads to inflammatory responses that may weaken the membranes, and stresses (fetal or maternal) that alter the fetal hypothalamic–pituitary–adrenal axis. Once preterm labour has begun, it is not possible to stop it for more than a few days. At-risk patients in early pregnancy may be given corticosteroids to enhance the development of fetal lung maturity or a tocolytic (IV magnesium sulfate) to stop contractions for a few days, and to allow for an opportunity to give steroids and prepare for preterm delivery. (Magnesium sulfate also reduces the risk of cerebral palsy in the neonate.)

POSTTERM PREGNANCY

Approximately 10% of all pregnancies are delivered at more than 14 days after the estimated date of delivery (or >280 days gestation, 42 weeks post last menstrual period [LMP]). In general, two situations may occur in postpartum pregnancies: the placenta may continue its normal functions and the fetus continues to grow resulting in fetal macrosomia (fetus >4000 g), or placental insufficiency occurs, resulting in a reduction of oxygenation and nutrition to the fetus. The latter situation is more common and leads to higher rates of fetal morbidity and mortality. Macrosomia may result in a more complicated delivery because of cephalopelvic disproportion, and possible traumatic birth, especially in infants greater than 5000 g. Postmaturity syndrome is found in about one-fifth of postterm deliveries and is related to placental insufficiency and arrested fetal growth (IUGR). The neonate with postmaturity syndrome has long fingernails, little subcutaneous fat, meconium staining and low weight.

If the clinical situation warrants induction of labour, the most common methods include artificial rupture of the membranes, stripping of the membranes (causing prostaglandin release), balloon dilation of the cervix, intravaginal prostaglandin E_2 and intravenous oxytocin infusion.

NEONATAL RESPIRATORY DISTRESS SYNDROME

Infants born prematurely are at high risk of respiratory distress syndrome (RDS), with the most common presenting symptoms being rapid, laboured breathing, and cyanosis shortly after birth. More than 95% of infants born at 22 to 24 weeks have RDS with the incidence dropping to about 5% in fetuses born 10 weeks later. Deficiency of pulmonary surfactant produces RDS, with other factors such as hypovolaemia and barotrauma adding to the pathophysiology. In RDS, the lungs are underinflated, and the alveoli contain a fluid with a high protein content that resembles a glassy, or hyaline, membrane (RDS was formerly referred to as hyaline membrane disease). This membrane is thought to be derived from a combination of substances in the circulation and from the injured pulmonary epithelium. It has been suggested that prolonged intrauterine asphyxia (impaired or absent exchange of oxygen and carbon dioxide) may produce irreversible changes in the type II alveolar cells, making them incapable of producing surfactant. Other factors such as sepsis, aspiration and pneumonia may inactivate surfactant, leading to an absence or deficiency of surfactant in premature and even some full-term infants. Maternal glucocorticoid treatment during pregnancy accelerates fetal lung development and surfactant production. Positive-pressure ventilation and other techniques (invasive and noninvasive) to maintain alveolar expansion are the main treatment modalities. Administration of exogenous surfactant (surfactant replacement therapy) reduces the severity of RDS and the chance of neonatal mortality.

Case Outcome

Neonatal blood glucose levels were 2.3 mmol/L at 6 hours and then 4.3 mmol/L at 8 hours. Cord gases were normal. All biochemical, genetic, immunological and infectious disease testing of the neonate were normal. Three years later, the child had 'caught up' in growth.

Additional reflections: Given the normal test results from the neonate, what might be the reason for the intrauterine growth retardation (IUGR)? Could this IUGR have been treated if it was detected earlier and what might that treatment have been? What long term (childhood and adult) impacts might IUGR have for this infant?

QUESTIONS

1. Relating to parturition, which of the following statements is correct?
   a. Labour is divided into two stages: cervical dilation and expulsion
   b. Oxytocin is administered clinically to prevent early labour
   c. The fetus produces relaxin to initiate uterine contractions and cervical dilation
   d. Contractions become less intense as the cervical canal dilates
   e. The formation of a haematoma, deep to the placenta, and myometrial contraction prevent excessive uterine bleeding

2. Which of the following statements is true related to the transition from fetal to neonatal life?
   a. Occurs gradually over about 2 to 3 hours as the fetal systems adapt to extrauterine life
   b. More than 25% of infants born require some assistance to begin breathing
   c. Fluid from the lungs of the newborn is primarily expelled from the mouth and often requires suctioning
   d. Clamping of the umbilical cord increases blood pressure in the neonate
   e. Delayed clamping of the umbilical cord may result in decreases in neonatal haemoglobin and iron stores and is not recommended

3. Which of the following is true related to intrauterine growth restriction (IUGR)?
   a. IUGR arises primarily from fetal causes, most often related to chromosomal defects
   b. IUGR is the leading cause of fetal and neonatal morbidity and mortality
   c. Symmetric pattern of biometric indices is required for a diagnosis of IUGR
   d. Once IUGR is suspected, serial examination by ultrasound can be discontinued
   e. Provided the infant survives the neonatal period, additional complications from IUGR are not common

BIBLIOGRAPHY

Committee on Obstetric Practice. Committee Opinion. American College of Obstetricians and Gynecologists 2017;684:1–6. (reaffirmed in 2018).

Fraser D. Newborn adaptation to extrauterine life. In: Simpson KR, Creehan PA, O'Brien-Abel N, et al. (Eds.). AWHONN's Perinatal Nursing. 5th ed. Philadelphia, PA: Wolters Kluwer; 2021. p. 581–96.

Jelin AC, Sagaser KG, Wilkins-Haug L. Prenatal genetic testing. Pediatr Clin North Am 2019;66:281–93.

Rhoades JS, Stout MJ, Woolfolk C, et al. Normal cervical effacement in term labor. Am J Perinatol 2019;36(1):034–8.

Sharma D. Golden hour of neonatal life: Need of the hour. Matern Health Neonatol Perinatol 2017;19(3):6.

Sharma D, Sharma P, Shastri S. Genetic, metabolic and endocrine aspect of intrauterine growth restriction: an update. J Matern Fetal Neonatal Med 2017;30(19):2263–75.

Van Vonderen JJ, Roest AAW, Siew M, Walther FJ, Hooper SB, te Pas AB. Measuring physiological changes during the transition to life after birth. Neonatology 2014;105:230–42.

SECTION 2

DEVELOPMENT OF ORGAN SYSTEMS

8 Development of the Cardiovascular, Haematopoietic and Lymphatic Systems

Case Scenario

FE is a 30-year-old female with a history of an open fracture of her left tibia and fibula; this trauma was the result of a bicycle–automobile collision. Three days after surgery to stabilise the fracture, FE developed a thrombus in her left popliteal vein. Twelve hours later, FE had acute confusion, right-sided facial paralysis and hemiplegia. Magnetic resonance imaging of her brain revealed the following:

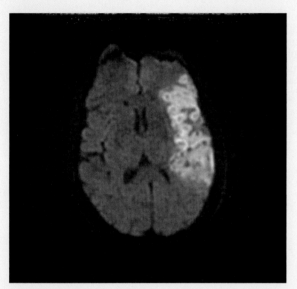

Fig. 8.1 Magnetic resonance image of the brain.

Questions for reflection: What are the possible complications of an open versus closed fracture? What might be the cause of the popliteal vein thrombus? What is the most likely cause of FE's neurological symptoms and the changes seen on the MRI? What congenital anomalies may have contributed to this neurological event?

DEVELOPMENT OF THE HEART

The heart, blood vessels and blood cells begin development early because of the rapidly increasing nutritional and oxygenation needs of the embryo, which can no longer be sustained by nutrient diffusion alone (see Video 8.1).

Mesodermal cells from the cranial portion of the primitive streak migrate to form a crescentic deposit of cardiac progenitor cells called the primary heart field and give rise to paired heart tubes. It appears that although these progenitor cells contribute to the formation of the heart tubes, they act principally as a scaffold for further development. Additional cardiac progenitor cells arise from the pharyngeal mesoderm, forming the second heart field, which is located medial and cranial to the first heart field. Second heart field cells appear to contribute to the ventricular myocardium and the myocardial wall of the outflow tract as well as drive the rapid growth and elongation of the heart tube (Fig. 8.3).

With lateral embryonic folding, the heart tubes fuse in a craniocaudal direction to form a single endocardial tube with three layers—myocardium (from splanchnic mesoderm), endocardium (epithelial cells) and intervening extracellular matrix (cardiac jelly). (Later in development, mesothelial cells of the sinus venosus [SV] spread over the myocardium to form the epicardium.) By day 21 the primordial heart starts to beat, and by day 24 it begins to transport blood. Early contractions occur in peristalsis-like waves and circulation is limited to an ebb-and-flow type, but by 28 days coordinated contractions result in a unidirectional flow. With cranial embryonic folding, the heart and pericardial cavity lie ventral to the foregut.

The elongation of the tubular heart during days 23 to 28 results in the formation of a sequential series of alternate dilations and constrictions: the bulbus cordis (composed of the truncus arteriosus, conus arteriosus and conus cordis), ventricle, atrium and SV (Fig. 8.4). The arterial and venous ends of the heart are fixed by the pharyngeal arches and septum transversum, respectively.

The truncus arteriosus is continuous cranially with the aortic sac from which the pharyngeal arch arteries arise (Fig. 8.5). The SV receives the umbilical, vitelline and common cardinal veins from the chorion, umbilical vesicle and embryo, respectively (Fig. 8.5).

During this heart configuration process, the endocardial tube undergoes dextral looping to form the bulboventricular loop, resulting in a primordial heart with its apex pointing to the left (Fig. 8.6). Bending of the heart tube also repositions the atrium and SV dorsal to the truncus arteriosus, bulbus cordis and ventricle. During bending, the SV develops right and left sinus horns. The heart then begins to invaginate into the pericardial cavity and is temporarily suspended from the dorsal wall by the dorsal mesocardium. As the central portion of the mesocardium undergoes apoptosis (forming the transverse pericardial sinus), the heart is now attached only at its cranial and caudal ends.

44

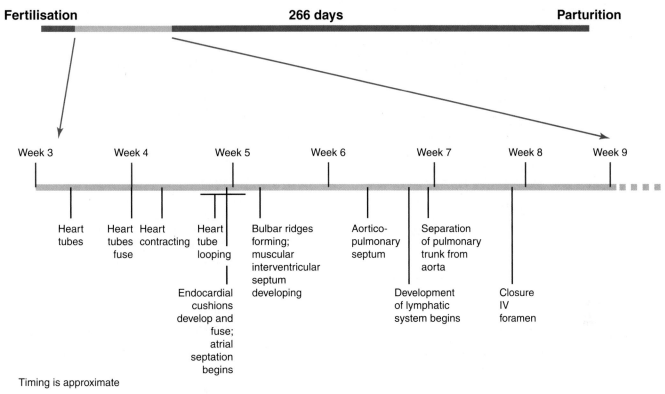

Fertilisation   **266 days**   **Parturition**

Week 3   Week 4   Week 5   Week 6   Week 7   Week 8   Week 9

Heart tubes

Heart tubes fuse

Heart contracting

Heart tube looping

Bulbar ridges forming; muscular interventricular septum developing

Aortico-pulmonary septum

Separation of pulmonary trunk from aorta

Endocardial cushions develop and fuse; atrial septation begins

Development of lymphatic system begins

Closure IV foramen

Timing is approximate

Fig. 8.2   Timeline of development related to the cardiovascular, hematopoietic and lymphatic systems.

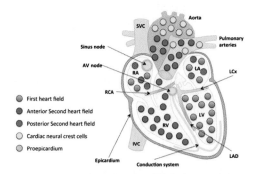

Fig. 8.3   Diagram of the contribution of heart fields to the developing heart. *AV,* Atrioventricular; *IVC,* inferior vena cava; *LAD, LCx, RCA,* right carotid artery; *RV,* right ventricle; *SVC,* superior vena cava. (From Kloesel B, DiNardo JA, Body SC. Cardiac embryology and molecular mechanisms of congenital heart disease – A Primer for Anesthesiologists. Anesth Analg 2016; 123(3): 551–569. Fig. 6.)

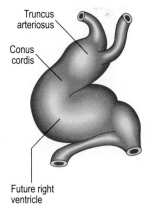

Fig. 8.4   Ventral view of the developing heart at approximately 35 days. (Modified from Mitchell B, Sharma R. *Embryology: An Illustrated Colour Text.* 2nd ed. London: Elsevier; 2009. Fig. 6.4.)

SEPTATION OF THE HEART

By about 31 days, partitioning of the atrioventricular (AV) canal, primordial atrium, ventricle and outflow tract, essentially concurrent processes, begins to take place and is completed by the beginning of the fetal period (start of week 9).

AV endocardial cushions form on the dorsal and ventral walls of the AV canal and proximal ventricular outflow tract, initially from both cardiac jelly and neural crest cells. During the fifth week, the cushions are invaded by mesenchymal cells derived by epithelial-to-mesenchymal transformation of endocardial cells. As the AV cushions grow, approach each other and fuse, the AV canal is separated into right and left canals, which partially separate the developing atrium and ventricle (Fig. 8.7).

ATRIA

By day 28, the septum primum begins to form from second heart field cells from the roof of the primordial atrium. The septum primum grows towards the fusing endocardial cushions, creating a partially divided common atrium (Fig. 8.7). The foramen primum remains between the free edge of the septum primum and the endocardial cushions, serving as a shunt for oxygenated blood to pass from the right to the left atrium. However, further growth of the septum primum results in gradual disappearance of the foramen primum as the mesenchymal cap of the septum primum fuses with AV endocardial cushions. Before the foramen primum disappears, however, perforations in the central part of the septum primum form and coalesce to create the foramen secundum

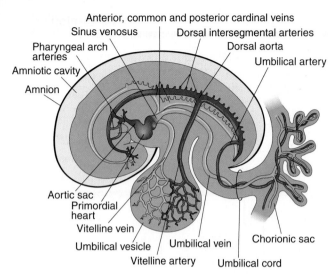

Fig. 8.5   Diagram of the early (approximately 26-day) cardiovascular system. (Modified Moore KL, Persaud TVN, Torchia MG. *The Developing Human: Clinically Oriented Embryology.* 10th ed. Philadelphia: Elsevier; 2015. Fig. 13.2.)

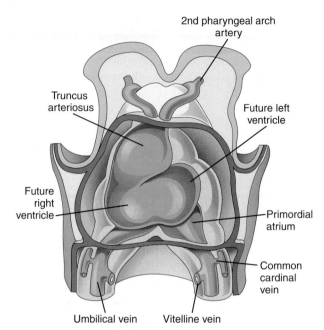

Fig. 8.6   Ventral view of the developing heart showing looping. (Modified from Moore KL, Persaud TVN, Torchia MG. *The Developing Human: Clinically Oriented Embryology.* 10th ed. Philadelphia: Elsevier; 2015. Fig. 13.7E.)

(Fig. 8.7), ensuring continued shunting of oxygenated blood. The septum secundum grows immediately adjacent to the septum primum, from the right atrial ventrocranial wall (Fig. 8.7). As this muscular septum grows, it overlaps the foramen secundum to form the foramen ovale, an incomplete partition between the atria. Over time, the cranial portion of the septum primum gradually disappears; the caudal portion, attached to the fused endocardial cushions, forms the flap-like valve of the foramen ovale. The foramen ovale shunts most of the oxygenated blood entering the right atrium (from the inferior vena cava [IVC]) to pass into the left atrium and also prevents flow in the opposite direction, as the septum primum closes against the septum secundum (Fig. 8.7).

VENTRICLES

Early septation of the primitive ventricle begins with the formation of the muscular interventricular septum from myocytes in the floor of the ventricle near its apex (Fig. 8.8). The growth of the muscular septum is attributed to both dilation of the ventricles on either side of its origin and proliferation of septal myoblasts. The interventricular foramen, which forms between the free edge of the interventricular septum and the fused endocardial cushions, allows connectivity between the right and left ventricles. The membranous (superior) part of the interventricular septum is derived from the endocardial cushions (right side) as well as neural crest cells of the outflow tract. Subsequent closure of the interventricular foramen results from the fusion of tissues from three sources: the right bulbar ridge, the left bulbar ridge and the endocardial cushion. The membranous interventricular septum merges with the aorticopulmonary septum (Fig. 8.8) and the muscular part of the interventricular septum. At completion of ventricular septation the pulmonary trunk and aorta connect with the right and left ventricle, respectively.

BULBUS CORDIS AND TRUNCUS ARTERIOSUS

Bulbar and truncal ridges form during the fifth week in the walls of the bulbus cordis and truncus arteriosus, respectively

(Fig. 8.9). These ridges are populated largely from mesenchyme of neural crest origin by way of the primordial pharynx and pharyngeal arches. As the ridges enlarge, they meet in the lumen creating the aorticopulmonary septum. The spiral orientation is believed to be caused in part by mechanical forces related to the streaming of blood from the ventricles. The septum results in the formation of two distinct lumens which will become the ascending aorta and pulmonary trunk. The remaining bulbus cordis is incorporated into the walls of the definitive ventricles as the conus arteriosus (infundibulum; right ventricle) and the walls of the aortic vestibule (left ventricle).

DEVELOPMENT OF CARDIAC VALVES

When partitioning of the truncus arteriosus is nearly completed the semilunar valves begin to develop from three swellings of subendocardial tissue around the orifices of the aorta and pulmonary trunk. These swelling are comprised of epicardial and neural crest cells and undergo morphological reshaping to form three thin-walled cusps. The tricuspid and mitral valves develop similarly from localised proliferations of tissue around the AV canals.

The ventricular walls undergo cavitation and form trabeculae carneae, some of which become papillary muscles and chordae tendineae. The cords run from the papillary muscles to the AV valves.

ATRIAL MORPHOGENESIS

The SV opens into the centre of the dorsal wall of the primordial atrium, and its right and left horns are similar in size. Owing to development of vessel and mechanical forces, the right horn becomes enlarged and its orifice shifts rightward and later becomes incorporated into the wall of the right atrium forming a smooth surface. The left horn of the SV becomes the coronary sinus. The remainder of the anterior internal surface of the atrial wall and the right auricle have a rough trabeculated appearance, and are derived from the primordial atrium. The smooth part and the rough part are demarcated by the crista terminalis and the sulcus terminalis. The small left auricle is derived from the primordial atrium; its internal surface has a rough trabeculated appearance.

The primordial pulmonary vein develops as an outgrowth of the dorsal atrial wall, just to the left of the septum primum. As the atrium enlarges, the primordial pulmonary

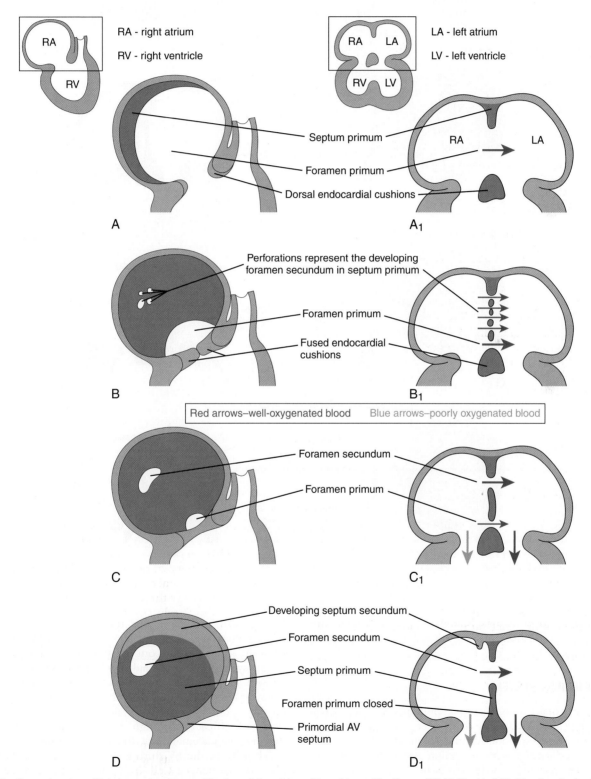

Fig. 8.7 Coronal and sagittal views showing partitioning of the atrium. (From Moore KL, Persaud TVN, Torchia MG. *The Developing Human: Clinically Oriented Embryology.* 10th ed. Philadelphia: Elsevier; 2015. Fig. 13.13.)

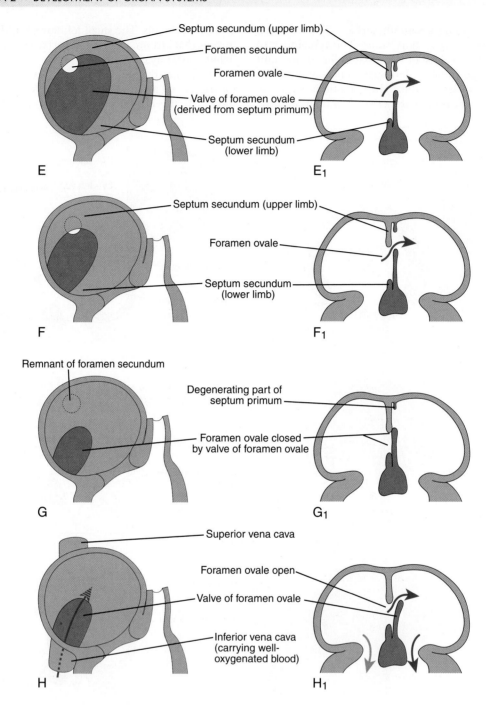

Fig. 8.7   (Cont.)

vein and its large pulmonary branches are incorporated into the atrial wall, forming the smooth walled part of the left atrium (Fig. 8.10).

CONDUCTING SYSTEM

In the early heart tube, myocytes spontaneously depolarise resulting in slow conduction of an electrical impulse. These cells have relatively poor contractile qualities because sarcomeres and sarcoplasmic reticulum are underdeveloped. The earliest pacemaker activity is found in the inflow (SV) and outflow (atrioventricular canal [AVC]) tracts, and this continues even with the addition of more cells during heart

tube growth, indicating that the added myocytes develop this pacemaker phenotype. The waves of contraction move from the inflow tract to outflow tract. Over time, two pools of myocytes develop; a small pool of pacemaker-like activity with slow conduction (SV and AVC), and the majority of myocytes (myocardium) in the atria and ventricles that quickly conduct the wave of depolarisation and contract with high efficacy. Although the primordial atrium acts as the interim pacemaker of the heart, the sinoatrial node develops from the SV during the fifth week and becomes the early pacemaker. Cells from the AVC form the AV node and bundle and split into right and left bundle branches. These branches are distributed throughout the ventricular

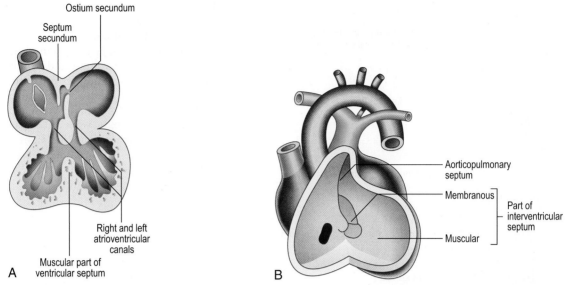

Fig. 8.8   (A) Coronal view of the heart showing partitioning of the ventricle. (B) Partitioning of the ventricles, bulbus cordis, and truncus arteriosus. (Modified from Mitchell B, Sharma R. *Embryology: An Illustrated Colour Text.* 2nd ed. London: Elsevier; 2009. Figs 6.5, 6.6C.)

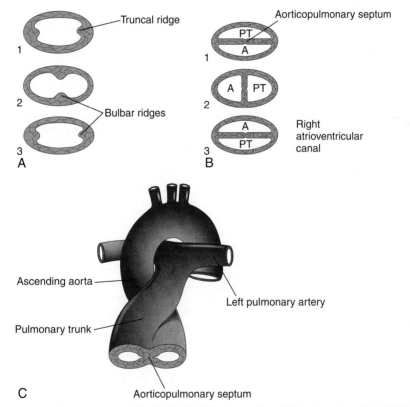

Fig. 8.9   Partitioning of the bulbus cordis and truncus arteriosus. (A, B) Cross section of the truncus arteriosus (1) and bulbus cordis (2,3) at 5 and 6 weeks, respectively. C. Final structure and position of the great arteries. *A,* Atrium; *PT,* pulmonary trunk. (Modified from Moore KL, Persaud TVN, Torchia MG. *The Developing Human: Clinically Oriented Embryology.* 10th ed. Philadelphia: Elsevier; 2015. Fig. 13.21B, E, H.)

myocardium. As the four chambers of the heart develop, a band of connective tissue grows in from the epicardium (visceral layer of the serous pericardium), subsequently separating the muscle of the atria from that of the ventricles, so that the conducting system is normally the only signal pathway from the atria to the ventricles. Although the sinoatrial and AV nodes and the AV bundle are richly invested by nerves, the conducting system is well developed before these nerves enter the heart.

VASCULAR SYSTEM

In a 4-week-old embryo, vitelline veins return poorly oxygenated blood from the umbilical vesicle, umbilical veins carry well-oxygenated blood from the chorionic sac and common cardinal veins return poorly oxygenated blood from the body of the embryo to the heart (see Video 8.2).

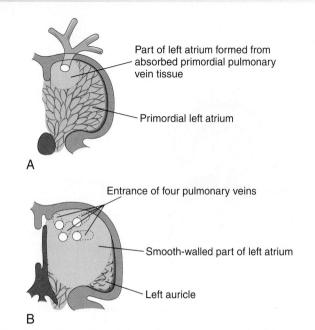

Fig. 8.10 Absorption of the pulmonary vein into the left atrium; (A) 5-6 weeks, (B) 8 weeks. (Modified from Moore KL, Persaud TVN, Torchia MG. *The Developing Human: Clinically Oriented Embryology.* 10th ed. Philadelphia: Elsevier; 2015. Fig. 13.16B, D.)

VENOUS

The vitelline paired veins follow the omphaloenteric duct, pass through the septum transversum and enter the SV. The left vitelline vein gradually undergoes apoptosis and the right forms most of the hepatic portal system, as well as a portion of the IVC. Initially, the umbilical veins pass on each side of the developing liver and carry well-oxygenated blood from the placenta to the SV. As the liver develops and increases in size, the umbilical veins empty directly into the liver. The right umbilical vein degenerates, leaving the left to carry well-oxygenated blood from the placenta to the embryo. The ductus venosus, a venous shunt, develops within the liver connecting the left umbilical vein with the IVC forming a bypass through the liver, enabling most of the blood from the placenta to pass directly to the heart without passing through the developing capillary network of the liver.

The anterior and posterior cardinal veins develop early (Fig. 8.11) and drain the cranial and caudal parts of the embryo, respectively. They join the common cardinal veins, which enter the SV. The anterior cardinal veins are interconnected by an anastomosis which shunts blood from the left to the right anterior cardinal vein—the shunt becomes the left brachiocephalic vein. The superior vena cava (SVC) forms from the right anterior cardinal vein and the right common cardinal vein. The posterior cardinal veins develop to support the mesonephroi with their only adult derivatives being the root of the azygos vein and common iliac veins. The subcardinal and supracardinal veins gradually develop to replace and supplement the posterior cardinal veins.

The subcardinal veins connect with each other through the subcardinal anastomosis, and with the posterior cardinal veins through the mesonephric sinusoids. The subcardinal

veins form the stem of the left renal vein, the suprarenal veins, the testicular and ovarian veins, and a portion of the IVC. Cranial to the kidneys, the supracardinal veins connect by an anastomosis that is represented in the adult by the azygos and hemiazygos veins. Caudal to the kidneys, the left supracardinal vein degenerates and the right supracardinal vein becomes the inferior part of the IVC. Overall, the IVC is composed of four main segments: hepatic segment (derived from the hepatic vein and hepatic sinusoids); prerenal segment (derived from the right subcardinal vein); renal segment (the subcardinal–supracardinal anastomosis); and postrenal segment (the right supracardinal vein) (Fig. 8.11).

ARTERIAL

The pharyngeal arches, through neural crest cell differentiation, form pharyngeal arteries during weeks 4 to 5. These arteries arise from the aortic sac and terminate in the dorsal aortae (Fig. 8.5) Initially, the paired dorsal aortae run through the entire length of the embryo, but later the caudal portions fuse to form a single lower thoracic/abdominal aorta. The right cranial portions of the dorsal aortae regresses and the left portion becomes the primordial aorta. Approximately 30 branches of the dorsal aorta carry blood to the somites and their derivatives. In the neck, these intersegmental arteries join to form bilateral the vertebral arteries. In the thorax, the intersegmental arteries persist as intercostal arteries. In the abdomen, all but the fifth pair are transformed into lumbar arteries; the fifth pair become the common iliac arteries. In the sacral region, the intersegmental arteries form the lateral sacral arteries.

The derivatives of or contributions from the paired pharyngeal arch arteries include:

- First pair—maxillary and external carotid arteries
- Second pair—stapedial arteries
- Third pair—common carotid and internal carotid arteries
- Fourth pair—part of the arch of the aorta, proximal right subclavian artery, right dorsal aorta, right seventh intersegmental artery
- Fifth pair—none; rudimentary vessels that degenerate
- Sixth pair—left pulmonary artery, ductus arteriosus, right pulmonary artery.

The ductus arteriosus is a shunt that allows most blood leaving the pulmonary trunk to bypass the lungs because oxygenation is not required in the fetus. This shunt also prevents right ventricular overload, given that the pulmonary vascular resistance is high in the fetus.

The unpaired ventral branches of the dorsal aorta supply the umbilical vesicle, allantois and chorion. The vitelline arteries pass to the umbilical vesicle and become incorporated into the developing gut. Three vitelline artery derivatives remain as the celiac arterial trunk, the superior mesenteric artery and the inferior mesenteric artery. The paired umbilical arteries pass through the connecting stalk and carry poorly oxygenated blood to the placenta. The proximal parts of these arteries become internal iliac and superior vesical arteries, whereas the distal parts become the medial umbilical ligaments.

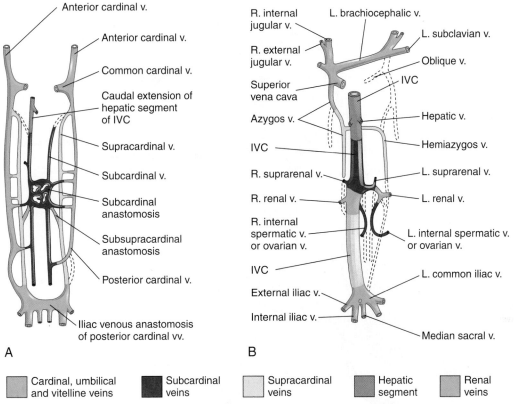

Fig. 8.11 Development of the main venous system of the fetus. (A) 7 weeks; (B) adult. *IVC,* Inferior vena cava. (Modified from Moore KL, Persaud TVN, Torchia MG. *The Developing Human: Clinically Oriented Embryology.* 10th ed. Philadelphia: Elsevier; 2015. Fig. 13.4B. D)

CIRCULATORY PATTERNS

EMBRYONIC

Blood enters the SV (Fig. 8.6) from the embryo (common cardinal veins), developing placenta (umbilical veins) and umbilical vesicle through the vitelline veins. From the SV, blood enters the primordial atrium and then passes through the AVC into the primordial ventricle. From the ventricle, blood is pumped through the bulbus cordis and truncus arteriosus into the aortic sac, from which it is distributed to the pharyngeal arch arteries in the pharyngeal arches. The blood then passes into the dorsal aortae for distribution to the embryo, umbilical vesicle and placenta.

FETAL

Highly oxygenated, nutrient-rich blood returns under high pressure from the placenta in the umbilical vein where approximately half of the blood passes directly into the ductus venosus to the IVC, bypassing the liver (Fig. 8.12). The remaining blood flows into the liver sinusoids and enters the IVC through the hepatic veins. Blood flow through the ductus venosus is regulated (physiological sphincter) to prevent overloading the heart when venous flow in the umbilical vein is high (e.g., during uterine contractions). Blood in the IVC from the umbilical vein mixes with poorly oxygenated blood in the IVC from the lower limbs, abdomen and pelvis. As a result, the blood entering the right atrium is not as well oxygenated as in the umbilical

vein. Most blood is then directed by the crista dividens through the foramen ovale and into the left atrium, where it mixes with a small amount of poorly oxygenated blood returning from the lungs through the pulmonary veins. The blood in the pulmonary veins has been deoxygenated by the metabolic needs of the lungs. From the left atrium the blood enters the left ventricle and leaves through the ascending aorta to the coronary arteries, neck, head and upper limbs.

The small amount of oxygenated blood that does not pass through the foramen ovale mixes with poorly oxygenated blood from the SVC and coronary sinus and passes into the right ventricle and the pulmonary trunk. Most of this blood passes through the ductus arteriosus into the descending aorta of the fetus and returns to the placenta through the umbilical arteries, whereas only a small percent of this blood flow goes to the lungs owing to high fetal pulmonary vascular resistance. The ductus arteriosus protects the lungs from circulatory overloading and allows the right ventricle to strengthen in preparation for functioning at full capacity at birth. Most of the blood in the descending aorta passes into the umbilical arteries and is returned to the placenta for reoxygenation, with the remaining blood suppling the viscera and the inferior part of the body.

TRANSITIONAL NEONATAL

Aeration of the lungs at birth is associated with a marked decrease in pulmonary vascular resistance, increase in pulmonary blood flow, and progressive thinning of the walls of

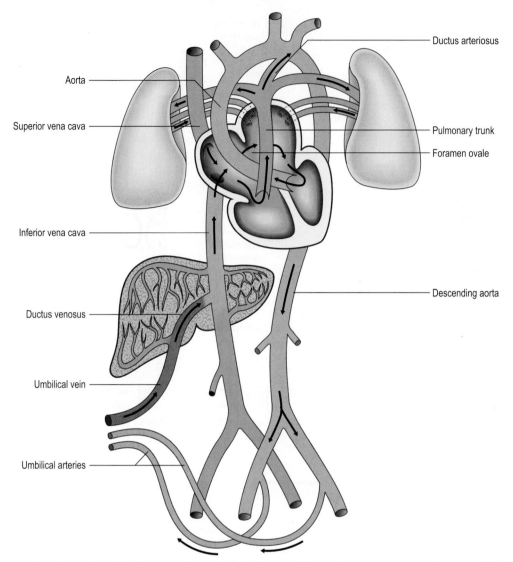

Aorta

Superior vena cava

Inferior vena cava

Ductus venosus

Umbilical vein

Umbilical arteries

Ductus arteriosus

Pulmonary trunk

Foramen ovale

Descending aorta

Fig. 8.12   Fetal circulation. (From Mitchell B, Sharma R. *Embryology: An Illustrated Colour Text.* 2nd ed. London: Elsevier; 2009. Fig. 6.15).

the pulmonary arteries because of stretching of the lungs. These changes, in combination with loss of flow from the umbilical cord, result in the pressure in the left atrium being higher than in the right and functional closure of the foramen ovale (Fig. 8.13). Blood from the right ventricle now passes easily through the pulmonary trunk for oxygenation in the lungs. With pulmonary vascular resistance now lower than the systemic vascular resistance, blood flow in the ductus arteriosus reverses, passing from the descending aorta to the pulmonary trunk.

The ductus arteriosus begins to close functionally at birth, but a small amount of blood may continue to be shunted from the aorta to the pulmonary trunk for 24 to 48 hours in a normal full-term neonate. When the pO_2 of the blood passing through the ductus arteriosus reaches approximately 50 mmHg, the wall of the ductus arteriosus constricts, mediated by the effects of prostaglandin E_2 secretion. In premature neonates and in those with persistent hypoxia the ductus arteriosus may remain open much longer.

At birth, the right ventricular wall is thicker than the left ventricular wall because the right ventricle has been working

harder in utero, but this difference in thickness reverses by the end of the first month.

DERIVATIVE OF FETAL BLOOD VESSELS AND SHUNTS

The umbilical vein remains patent for a considerable period in the neonate and may be cannulated for venous access. The intraabdominal part of the umbilical vein eventually becomes the round ligament of the liver passing from the umbilicus to the porta hepatis and is attached to the left branch of the portal vein. The ductus venosus becomes the ligamentum venosum passing through the liver from the left branch of the portal vein and attaching to the IVC. Most of the intraabdominal parts of the umbilical arteries become medial umbilical ligaments although the proximal parts remain as the superior vesical arteries. The foramen ovale undergoes anatomic closure by about the third month. The septum primum forms the floor of the oval fossa whereas the inferior edge of the septum secundum forms the limbus fossa ovalis marking the former boundary of the foramen

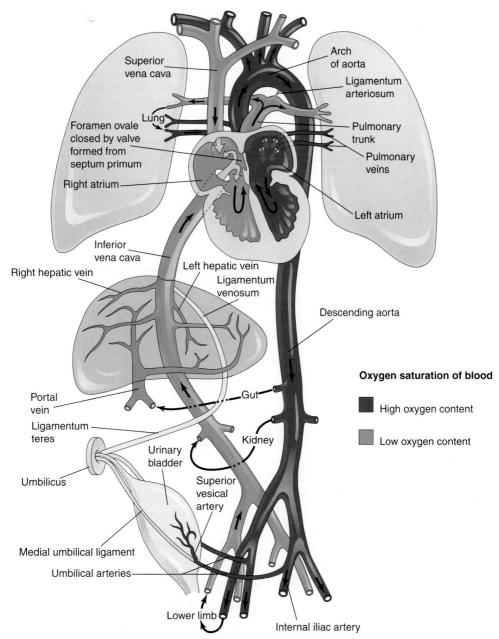

Fig. 8.13 Neonatal circulation. (From Moore KL, Persaud TVN, Torchia MG. *The Developing Human: Clinically Oriented Embryology.* 10th ed. Philadelphia: Elsevier; 2015. Fig. 13.47).

ovale. Functional closure of the ductus arteriosus is usually completed within the first few days after birth, with anatomic closure occurring about 3 to 4 months later, becoming the ligamentum arteriosum extending from the left pulmonary artery to the arch of the aorta.

HAEMATOGENESIS

Blood cells develop from specialised endothelial cells (hemangiogenic epithelium) of vessels as they grow on the umbilical vesicle and allantois at the end of the third week. Progenitor blood cells also arise directly from hemangiopoietic stem cells. Haematogenesis does not begin within the embryo proper until the fifth week. It occurs first along the

aortic–gonad–mesonephros region (dorsal aorta and urogenital ridges), and then in various parts of the embryonic mesenchyme, mainly the liver. Haematogenesis later occurs in the spleen, bone marrow and lymph nodes. Fetal and adult erythrocytes are derived from haematopoietic progenitor cells.

DEVELOPMENT OF THE LYMPHATIC SYSTEM

Precursor endothelial cells of the lymphatic vessels are derived from the cardinal veins. The lymphatic vessels develop using similar mechanism (e.g., lymphangiogenesis) as blood vessels with the newly developed lymphatic capillaries

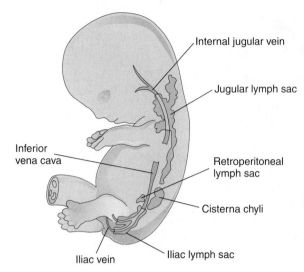

Fig. 8.14 Primary lymph sacs in embryo between the seventh and eighth weeks. From Moore KL, Persaud TVN, & Torchia MG. *The Developing Human: Clinically Oriented Embryology.* 10th ed. Philadelphia: Elsevier; 2015. Fig. 13.54.)

joining each other to form a network and ultimately connect with the venous system. Lymphatic vessels then connect to lymph sacs (Fig. 8.14), future locations of lymph nodes. From the sacs, vessels traverse parallel to the main veins to the head, neck and upper limbs (jugular lymph sacs); veins of the lower trunk and lower limbs (iliac lymph sacs); and primordial gut (retroperitoneal lymph sac and the cisterna chyli). Two larger channels (right and left thoracic ducts) connect the jugular lymph sacs with the cisterna chyli and interconnect through an anastomosis. The thoracic duct is ultimately formed by the caudal right thoracic duct, the anastomosis and the cranial left thoracic duct, with many variations. The right lymphatic duct is derived from the cranial part of the right thoracic duct. The thoracic duct and right lymphatic duct connect with the venous system at the venous angle between the internal jugular vein and subclavian vein.

Mesenchymal cell invasion transforms the lymph sacs into groups of lymph nodes. The original cavity of the lymph sacs becomes the lymph sinuses. Mesenchymal cells also produce the lymph node capsule and connective tissue. Peyer's patches, small intestine lymphoid tissue, begin to develop at approximately 15 weeks.

Three of the four tonsil groups develop from adjacent aggregations of lymph nodules:

- tubal tonsils—aggregations at the pharyngeal openings of the pharyngotympanic tubes
- pharyngeal tonsils—aggregations in the nasopharyngeal wall
- lingual tonsils—aggregations in the root of the tongue

The palatine tonsils develop from the endoderm of the second pharyngeal pouches and nearby mesenchyme.

The spleen develops from mesenchymal cells in the dorsal mesogastrium. Lymph nodules also develop in the mucosa of the respiratory and alimentary systems.

Molecular Biology Considerations

- Pitx2c, BMP, Notch, Wnt and SHH pathways—left–right patterning of the heart tube and cardiac looping
- TGF-β_1 and TGF-β_2, BMP2A and BMP4, Slug, ChALK2, GPCR signalling—cardiac epithelial to mesenchymal transformation and formation of the endocardial cushions
- Notch and Runx1—regulating haematopoietic stem cells and endothelial-to-haematopoietic transition, respectively
- LYVE1 and VEGFR3—delineate progenitor endothelial cells
- Prox1, Sox18 and COUP-TF11—migration and proliferation of precursor lymphatic cells
- LTi—trafficking of lymphatic endothelial cells, primary lymphoid tissue organiser (LTo)

CLINICAL ISSUES

VENTRICULAR SEPTAL DEFECT

Ventricular septal defects (VSDs) are the most common congenital heart defect (CHD) (25% of all CHDs) although 30% to 50% close spontaneously during the first 12 months postpartum.

If tissue from the right side of the endocardial cushion does not proliferate and fuse with the aorticopulmonary septum and the muscular part of the interventricular septum, the membranous portion of the interventricular septum will not be formed. This results in incomplete closure of the interventricular foramen and creates the most common VSD. Alternatively, if the muscular part of the interventricular septum either does not grow or grows with defects, a muscular VSD results. Sometimes there are multiple small defects, producing what is sometimes called the 'Swiss cheese' VSD. Extremely rarely there is a complete absence of the interventricular septum resulting in a single ventricle or three-chambered heart.

ATRIAL SEPTAL DEFECTS

The most clinically important types of atrial septal defect (ASD) are:

- Ostium secundum (a defect in the area of the oval fossa)—resulting from defects of the septum primum and septum secundum. These are generally well tolerated into adulthood but may result in adult consequences such as pulmonary hypertension. Multiple defects may occur; defects of 2 cm or more in diameter are not uncommon.
- Endocardial cushion defects with ostium primum ASD—a deficiency of the endocardial cushions and the AV septum may result in a number of uncommon pathological configurations. The septum primum cannot fuse with the endocardial cushions and commonly there is a cleft in the anterior cusp of the mitral valve. In a complete type of endocardial cushion and AV septal defects, fusion of the endocardial cushions fails to occur, with a resultant central large AV septal defect (this occurs in approximately 20% of persons with Down syndrome).

- SV (high) ASDs—incomplete absorption of the SV into the right atrium and/or abnormal development of the septum secundum results in a deficiency in the superior part of the interatrial septum close to the entry of the SVC. It is commonly associated with partial anomalous pulmonary venous connections.

PATENT FORAMEN OVALE

In some situations, the valve of the foramen ovale is incompetent (patent foramen ovale [PFO]). When this occurs in isolation, it is not considered an ASD and usually has no haemodynamic impact. However, other concomitant heart defects (e.g., pulmonary stenosis) may cause an increase in right atrial pressure, leading to right-to-left shunting through the PFO and cyanosis. There may be circumstances (e.g., mitral valve stenosis) where the left atrial pressure is high, leading to left-to-right shunting, if the PFO is sufficiently incompetent. A probe PFO, with normal valve competence, exists in up to 25% of people. Although a PFO usually requires no treatment, cases of paradoxical embolism and PFO are reported amongst patients with cryptogenic stroke.

TETRALOGY OF FALLOT

Tetralogy of Fallot consists of four cardiac defects: pulmonary artery stenosis, ventricular septal defect, dextroposition of the aorta and right ventricular hypertrophy. In these cases the pulmonary trunk is also usually small. Cyanosis may or may not be present at birth depending on the severity of the defects. Tetralogy of Fallot results when division of the truncus arteriosus is unequal and the pulmonary trunk is stenotic; however, the aetiology of these changes is not well understood, although it is associated with DiGeorge syndrome (22q11.2 deletion syndrome). Primary surgical repair within the first year is the treatment of choice, although in some extreme situations a two-stage repair may be required.

TRANSPOSITION OF THE GREAT ARTERIES

If the aorticopulmonary septum does not spiral during partitioning of the bulbus cordis and truncus arteriosus, transposition of the great arteries (TGA) arises. The anatomical result has the aorta anterior and to the right of the pulmonary trunk, arising from the right ventricle; the pulmonary trunk arises from the left ventricle. Functionally, the result is that deoxygenated systemic venous blood returns to the right atrium, enters the right ventricle and then the aorta, passing to the body. Oxygenated blood via the pulmonary vein passes through the left ventricle and back into the pulmonary circulation. TGA is one cause of neonatal cyanotic heart disease and may be associated with ASD and VSD; if a PFO exists and there is patency of the ductus arteriosus, there is some mixing of oxygenated and deoxygenated blood. Definitive surgical correction is required; however a balloon atrial septoplasty may be a palliative step to permit blood to flow from left to right. One possible cause of TGA is a defective migration of neural crest cells to the bulbar and truncal ridges.

HYPOPLASTIC LEFT HEART SYNDROME

In these cases, in addition to the severe left ventricular hypoplasia, there is atresia or stenosis of the aortic and mitral valves, hypoplasia of the ascending aorta and aortic coarctation. As such, the right ventricle maintains both pulmonary and systemic circulations, the latter from blood passing through the ductus arteriosus and the foramen ovale. While in utero, and with pulmonary vascular resistance high, there is typically no consequence to the fetus. However, shortly after birth, as the ductus arteriosus closes, severe hypoperfusion occurs. The atrial septum will remain open and can allow for blood mixing. It is not uncommon for these infants to also have neurological anomalies. Prostaglandin E_2 is given to the neonate to maintain the patency of the ductus arteriosus. Surgical palliation (cardiac transplantation or a triple staged surgery [Norwood palliation]) is possible, with most children surviving into adulthood.

COARCTATION OF THE AORTA

Juxtaductal coarctations, those distal to the origin of the left subclavian artery at the entrance of the ductus arteriosus, are the most common (90%) and are associated with a bicuspid mitral valve in more than 70% of cases. The remainder of cases consists of postductal coarctation permitting development of a collateral circulation during the fetal period or preductal coarctation, where, in the fetus, blood flows through the ductus arteriosus to the descending aorta for distribution to the lower body. In severe coarctations, closure of the ductus arteriosus results in hypoperfusion and rapid deterioration. Prostaglandin E_2 is given to the neonate to maintain the patency of the ductus arteriosus and provide adequate blood flow to the lower limbs. The cause of aortic coarctation may be incorporation of ductus tissue into aorta (which is then reactive to oxygenation and constricts) or abnormal involution of a small segment of the left dorsal aorta.

AORTIC STENOSIS

There are three types of aortic stenosis with the most common (valvular stenosis) being thickening of the leaflets with some fusion of the commissures, to form a dome with a narrow opening. In subaortic (subvalvular) stenosis, there is often a band of fibrous tissue just inferior to the aortic valve. The narrowing of the aorta results from persistence of tissue that normally degenerates as the valve forms. Supravalvular aortic stenosis, the least common type, can be associated with other congenital defects in Williams syndrome. Severe aortic stenosis can quickly result in low cardiac output attributed to left ventricular failure whereas in less severe forms (bicuspid aortic valve) there may be no symptoms in childhood.

OTHER CARDIAC DEFECTS

PERSISTENT TRUNCUS

Persistent truncus refers to failure of the truncal ridges and the aorticopulmonary septum to develop and divide the truncus arteriosus into the aorta and pulmonary trunk, leaving a single truncus arteriosus which arises from the heart and supplies the systemic, pulmonary and coronary circulations. A VSD is always present.

EBSTEIN ANOMALY

Ebstein anomaly is a form of tricuspid valve dysplasia where at least one leaflet is displaced towards the apex resulting in some degree of loss of anterograde flow. Tethering of the leaflet(s) may also occur, as well as obstruction of the right ventricular outflow tract and other cardiac anomalies.

TRICUSPID ATRESIA

Tricuspid atresia occurs when a solid plate of tissue rather than the normal tricuspid valve develops, resulting in no communication between right atrium and right ventricle. Associated cardiac anomalies include ASD, VSD, AV septal defects and TGA.

VENA CAVAL ANOMALIES

The formation of the SVC and IVC is complex and many variations of these vessels are seen including:

- interrupted IVC—blood drains from the lower limbs, abdomen, and pelvis to the heart through the azygos system of veins;
- double SVC—persistent left SVC that opens into the right atrium through the coronary sinus;
- left SVC—blood from the right side is carried by the brachiocephalic vein to the left SVC, which empties into the coronary sinus;
- absent hepatic segment of the IVC—blood from inferior parts of the body drains into the right atrium through the azygos and hemiazygos veins; and
- double IVC—inferior part of the left supracardinal vein persists as a second IVC.

ANOMALOUS PULMONARY VENOUS CONNECTION

In these cases, none of the pulmonary veins connect with the left atrium. Most commonly (55%) a confluenced pulmonary vein connects with the innominate vein, the SVC, and then the right atrium. Other variations include the confluence vein descending below the diaphragm and emptying into the hepatic venous system, IVC and right atrium (compression of the vein by the diaphragm can occur leading to extremis); confluence entering the coronary sinus or directly into the right atrium; or, very rarely, where some of the veins enter the right atrium while others enter the right atrium. When obstruction does not occur and shunting happens through the foramen ovale, the neonate may be asymptomatic and elective surgery is indicated; symptomatic neonates will require urgent surgery.

CYSTIC HYGROMA

Large single or multilocular fluid-filled cavities in the inferolateral part of the neck are derived from lymphatic malformation, commonly from parts of a jugular lymph sac that are pinched off or from lymphatic spaces that fail to connect with the main lymphatic channels. Cystic hygromas are often diagnosed in utero by ultrasound and are commonly associated with aneuploidies, especially monosomy X. When the cystic hygroma is associated with general fetal oedema, the prognosis is poor.

Case Outcome

Magnetic resonance imaging revealed a thrombus in the main stem of the left middle cerebral artery. This was thought to be the result of a paradoxical embolism. Transthoracic echocardiography demonstrated a patent foramen ovale (PFO).

Additional reflections: Define and compare paradoxical embolism and cryptogenic stroke. What is the developmental cause of a PFO? What other cardiac defects put adult patients at risk for this type of stroke? Why would any of these defects not been detected at birth or in childhood? What are the implications of congenital heart anomalies in general, for adults?

QUESTIONS

1. Closure of the foramen primum results from fusion of the:
   a. septum primum and septum secundum
   b. septum secundum and the endocardial cushions
   c. septum primum and the endocardial cushions
   d. septum primum and the primordial pulmonary vein
   e. septum secundum and the membranous portion of the ventricular septum

2. Regarding the formation of the venous component of the vascular system:
   a. The vitelline veins are paired and enter the sinus venosus
   b. The umbilical veins carry poorly oxygenated blood to the sinus venosus
   c. The ductus venosus allows a portion of the blood flow to temporarily pass through the liver
   d. The superior vena cava forms mostly from the left anterior and common cardinal veins
   e. The inferior vena cava is comprised of two main segments, derived from the subcardinal vein

3. Which of the following is true related to the fetal cardiovascular system?
   a. The right ventricular wall is thicker than the left ventricular wall
   b. Blood flow is not controlled in the ductus venosus leading to increased flow during labour contractions as the umbilical cord is squeezed
   c. The ductus arteriosus remains closed until the first breath
   d. The umbilical vein closes very quickly after birth to balance blood flow
   e. The foramen ovale requires a few days for anatomical closure to occur

4. Regarding cardiac anomalies, which of the following statements is correct?
   a. In trisomy 21, the most common cardiac defect is the ostium secundum (a defect in the oval fossa area)
   b. Many ventricular septal defects found at birth close without treatment by about 12 months of age

c. Tetralogy of Fallot is a cyanotic defect that results from enlargement of the pulmonary trunk

d. Coarctation of the aorta almost always occurs well distant to the entrance of the ductus arteriosus

e. It is unusual for persistent truncus to occur with a simultaneous ventricular septal defect

BIBLIOGRAPHY

B. Kloesel, J.A. DiNardo, S.C. Body, Cardiac embryology and molecular mechanisms of congenital heart disease – A. Primer for Anesthesiologists, Anesth Analg 123 (3) (2016) 551–569.

A. Medvinsky, S. Rybtsov, S. Taoudi, Embryonic origin of the adult hematopoietic system: advances and questions, Development 138 (2011) 1017–1031.

T. Moore-Morris, P.P. Van Vliet, G. Andelfinger, M. Puceat, Role of epigenetics in cardiac development and congenital diseases, Physiol Rev 98 (2018) 2453–2475.

C.G. Nebigil, L. Desaubry, The role of GPCR signaling in cardiac epithelial to mesenchyml transformation (EMT), Trend Cardio Med 29 (4) (2019) 200–204.

R.J. Tomanek, Developmental progression of the coronary vasculature in human embryos and fetuses, Anat Rec 299 (2016) 25–41.

J.H. Van Weerd, V.M. Christoffels, The formation and function of the cardiac conduction system, Development 143 (2016) 197–210.

9 Development of the Body Cavities, Diaphragm, Respiratory System, and Head and Neck

Case Scenario

A 3-year-old boy (HD) was brought to his family physician by his mother. The major concern was a severe cold with rhinorrhoea and cough. That morning the mother had also noticed swelling on the left side of HD's neck. On examination, a mass measuring 2 cm × 2 cm was felt in the submandibular region. A course of antibiotics was prescribed for presumed lymphadenitis. HD has no significant past medical history.

Six days later, HD was brought to the local emergency department by his mother. Although his upper respiratory symptoms had decreased significantly, HD's mother was concerned that the left neck mass seemed to be increasing in size. On examination, the mass was now 3.5 cm × 3.5 cm. Further testing was ordered.

Questions for reflection: What are the most common causes of neck masses in children? In adults? What specific questions would you ask about HD's past medical history? How might the previous respiratory illness be related? What additional tests would be helpful toward establishing a diagnosis?

DEVELOPMENT OF BODY CAVITIES

Intraembryonic mesoderm is formed by cells derived from the epiblast and primitive streak. During the third week, three regions of mesoderm can be distinguished between the layers of ectoderm and endoderm: paraxial, intermediate and lateral mesoderm (Fig. 9.2). The paraxial mesoderm undergoes condensation and divides to form the somites, precursors of the musculoskeletal system. The intermediate mesoderm contributes to the urogenital and other systems. The lateral mesoderm is continuous with the extraembryonic mesoderm covering the umbilical vesicle and amnion (see Video 9.1).

The primordium of the embryonic body cavities begins as isolated coelomic spaces that develop in the lateral intraembryonic mesoderm, which then coalesce into the horseshoe-shaped intraembryonic coelom. The cranial curved portion of the intraembryonic coelom will become the pericardial cavity, whereas the paired lateral components will become the pleural and peritoneal cavities. The coelom divides the lateral mesoderm into two components: the somatic (parietal) lateral mesoderm, continuous with the extraembryonic mesoderm covering the amnion, and the splanchnic (visceral) lateral mesoderm continuous with the extraembryonic mesoderm covering the umbilical vesicle (Fig. 9.3). During embryonic folding, the somatic mesoderm and overlying ectoderm form the somatopleure (body wall), whereas the splanchnic mesoderm and underlying endoderm form splanchnopleure (the embryonic gut). Lateral folding also causes the limbs of the coelom to be positioned together on the ventral aspect of the embryo, remaining connected to the extraembryonic coelom. This connection is lost at approximately week 11 when the physiological intestinal hernia is reduced (Fig. 9.4; see also Fig. 11.4)

The intraembryonic coelom becomes divided into three regions in the fourth week: a pericardial cavity, two pericardioperitoneal canals and a peritoneal cavity (Fig. 9.5). The pericardioperitoneal canals lie lateral to the proximal foregut and dorsal to the septum transversum, the primordium of the central tendon of the diaphragm. The walls of the cavities are lined by mesothelium (epithelium) derived from the somatic and splanchnic mesoderm, forming the parietal and visceral walls and associated peritoneum.

Early lung development occurs simultaneously with the development of the body cavities. The bronchial buds (primordia of bronchi and lungs) grow into the pericardioperitoneal canals creating folds in the lateral wall of each canal. The created pleuroperitoneal folds are then located superior to the developing lungs, and the pleuroperitoneal folds are located inferior to the lungs (Fig. 9.6). As the folds enlarge, they form pleuropericardial and pleuroperitoneal membranes that delineate and separate the pericardial cavity from pleural cavities, and separate the pleural cavities from the peritoneal cavity, respectively. The pleuropericardial membranes fuse with the mesenchyme ventral to the oesophagus and form the primordial mediastinum, a mass of mesenchyme that extends from the sternum to the vertebral column and separates the developing lungs (Fig. 9.7). As the lungs grow and the pleural cavities expand ventrally around the heart, they extend into the body wall, splitting the mesenchyme into two layers: the thoracic wall and the fibrous pericardium (Fig. 9.7) The pleuroperitoneal membranes extend ventromedially until they fuse with the dorsal mesentery of the oesophagus and septum transversum (Fig. 9.8). Complete closure requires the migration of myoblasts into the pleuroperitoneal membranes.

DEVELOPMENT OF THE DIAPHRAGM

The diaphragm develops from four components: the septum transversum, the pleuroperitoneal membranes, the dorsal mesentery of oesophagus and muscular ingrowth from lateral body walls.

The septum transversum, comprised of mesodermal tissue, grows from the ventrolateral body wall, and initially separates the heart from the liver, with a large part of the

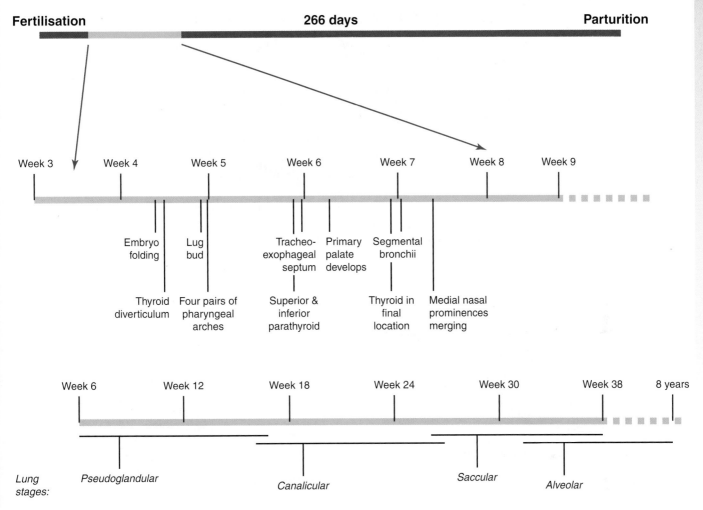

Fig. 9.1   Timeline of development related to body cavities, diaphragm, respiratory system and the head and neck.

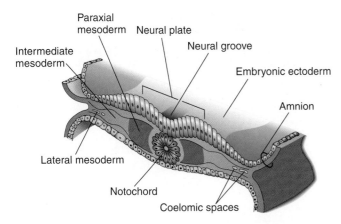

Fig. 9.2   Transverse section of the embryo at approximately 18 days. (Modified from Moore KL, Persaud TVN, & Torchia, MG. *The Developing Human: Clinically Oriented Embryology*. 10th ed. Philadelphia: Elsevier; 2015. Fig. 14.1B.)

developing liver initially embedded in the septum. With head folding and growth of the lungs, the septum fuses with the dorsal mesentery of the oesophagus and pleuroperitoneal membranes and forms an incomplete connective tissue partition between the thoracic and abdominal cavities (the primordial diaphragm). The septum transversum will become the central tendon of diaphragm. Over time the pleuroperitoneal membranes involute and represent only a small part of the final diaphragm. The dorsal mesentery of the oesophagus also fuses with the septum transversum and pleuroperitoneal membranes and contributes to the median portion of the diaphragm. Myoblasts invade the dorsal mesentery, producing the crura of the diaphragm. Myoblasts that differentiate from the mesenchyme in the septum transversum extend into the other diaphragm components and become the skeletal muscle of the diaphragm (Fig. 9.9). Muscular ingrowth from the lateral body wall contributes to the peripheral parts of the diaphragm. Lung growth and expansion of the thoracic cavity create the costodiaphragmatic recesses and the dome-like physical structure of the diaphragm (Fig. 9.10).

Myoblasts from the third to fifth cervical somites also migrate to the developing diaphragm. This migration includes the associated nerve fibres from the ventral primary rami of the third to fifth cervical spinal nerves. The myoblasts and nerves pass through the pleuropericardial membranes. The three pairs of nerve twigs join to form the phrenic nerve, supplying the motor innervation to the diaphragm. In addition, sensory fibres to the surfaces of the right and left

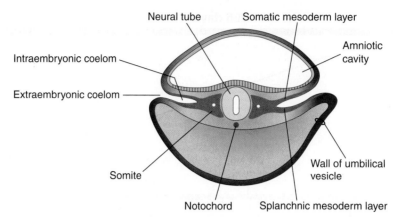

Fig. 9.3   Transverse section of the embryo at approximately 22 days. (Modified from Moore KL, Persaud TVN, & Torchia, MG. *The Developing Human: Clinically Oriented Embryology.* 10th ed. Philadelphia: Elsevier; 2015. Fig. 8.1B.)

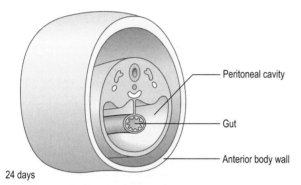

24 days

Fig. 9.4   Transverse section of the embryo at approximately 24 days. (Modified from Mitchell B, Sharma R. *Embryology: An Illustrated Colour Text.* 2nd ed. London: Elsevier; 2009. Fig. 1.13C.)

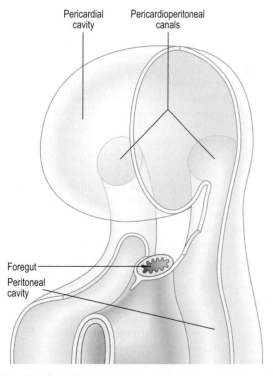

Fig. 9.5   Drawing of the lateral view of the embryo at 24 days. (From Mitchell B, Sharma R. *Embryology: An Illustrated Colour Text.* 2nd ed. London: Elsevier; 2009. Fig. 3.2.)

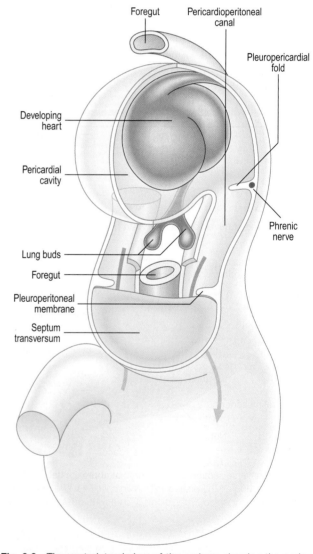

Fig. 9.6   The ventrolateral view of the embryo showing the pericardial cavity, pericardioperitoneal canals and their associated folds and membranes with surrounding tissues removed. (From Mitchell B, Sharma R. *Embryology: An Illustrated Colour Text.* 2nd ed. London: Elsevier; 2009. Fig. 3.4.)

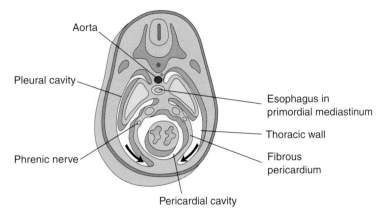

Fig. 9.7   Transverse section of the embryo at approximately week 7. (Modified from Moore KL, Persaud TVN, & Torchia, MG. *The Developing Human: Clinically Oriented Embryology.* 10th ed. Philadelphia: Elsevier; 2015. Fig. 8.5C.)

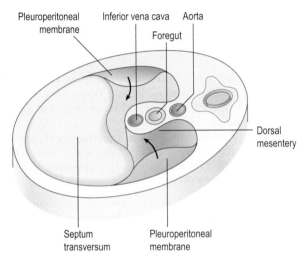

Fig. 9.8   Transverse section of the embryo at approximately week 6. (From Mitchell B, Sharma R. *Embryology: An Illustrated Colour Text.* 2nd ed. London: Elsevier; 2009. Fig. 3.5A.)

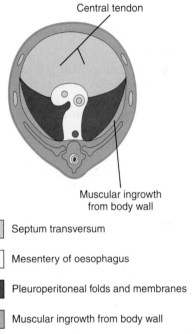

Septum transversum

Mesentery of oesophagus

Pleuroperitoneal folds and membranes

Muscular ingrowth from body wall

Fig. 9.9   Transverse section of the embryo at approximately week 12. (Modified from Moore KL, Persaud TVN, & Torchia, MG. *The Developing Human: Clinically Oriented Embryology.* 10th ed. Philadelphia: Elsevier; 2015. Fig. 8.7D.)

domes of the diaphragm are also provided by the phrenic nerves. As the length of the embryo continues to increase, the relative position of the diaphragm becomes more caudal. The dorsal portion of the diaphragm is found at the first lumbar vertebra, and the phrenic nerves grow correspondingly longer (approximately 30 cm long in adults). The contribution of the lateral body wall to the costal border of the diaphragm results in sensory fibres from the lower intercostal nerves innervating the costal border of the diaphragm.

RESPIRATORY SYSTEM

During week 4, the laryngotracheal groove appears in the anterior foregut, caudal to the fourth pharyngeal pouches (Fig. 9.11A) and within days forms the laryngotracheal diverticulum or lung bud (Fig. 9.11B). The diverticulum becomes invested with splanchnic mesenchyme that will form the connective tissue, cartilage and smooth muscle in the respiratory system. The endodermal lining of the laryngotracheal diverticulum forms the pulmonary epithelium and respiratory system glands. By the end of the fifth week, separation of the respiratory from the alimentary systems occurs when tracheoesophageal folds develop in the diverticulum and fuse to form the tracheoesophageal septum. From the

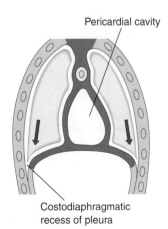

Fig. 9.10   Frontal section of the embryo. (Modified from Moore KL, Persaud TVN, & Torchia, MG. *The Developing Human: Clinically Oriented Embryology.* 10th ed. Philadelphia: Elsevier; 2015. Fig. 8.8B.)

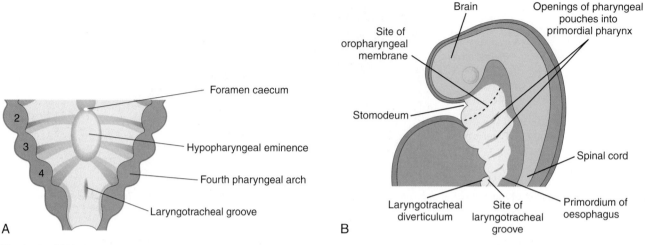

Fig. 9.11   (A) Horizontal section of the embryo at 4 weeks. (B) Sagittal section of the embryo at 4 weeks old. (Modified from Moore KL, Persaud TVN, & Torchia, MG. *The Developing Human: Clinically Oriented Embryology.* 10th ed. Philadelphia: Elsevier; 2015. Figs 10.4A, 10.1B.)

single diverticulum, right and left primary bronchial buds branch and grow into the pericardioperitoneal canals; later, secondary (Fig. 9.12A) and tertiary buds develop, continuing to expand the primordial lung size and the thoracic cavity (see Video 9.2).

Similarly, the connections to the bronchial buds enlarge and form the primordia of the main bronchi, which later subdivide into secondary bronchi with lobar, segmental and intrasegmental branches (Fig. 9.12B). The segmental bronchi, 10 in the right lung and 8 or 9 in the left lung, together with the surrounding mesenchyme form the bronchopulmonary segments. Approximately 17 orders of branches are formed by week 24 and respiratory bronchioles have developed. An additional seven orders of airways develop after birth.

The lungs develop through four overlapping stages with cranial segments maturing faster than caudal ones. These stages are classified by the microscopic appearance of the developing structures (Fig. 9.13):

- Pseudoglandular (5–17 weeks)—resembling tubuloacinar gland structure with all major pulmonary elements present except those involved with gas exchange. The first 20

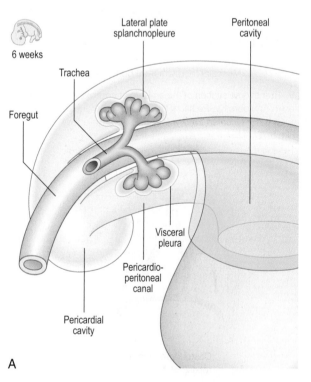

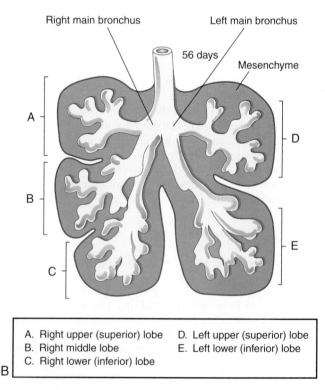

A. Right upper (superior) lobe	D. Left upper (superior) lobe
B. Right middle lobe	E. Left lower (inferior) lobe
C. Right lower (inferior) lobe	

Fig. 9.12   Drawing of the developing lungs showing (A) the division of the primary bronchial buds into secondary lung buds and (B) remaining subdivisions. (Modified from Mitchell B, Sharma R. *Embryology: An Illustrated Colour Text.* 2nd ed. London: Elsevier; 2009. Fig. 5.2 and Moore KL, Persaud TVN, & Torchia, MG. *The Developing Human: Clinically Oriented Embryology.* 10th ed. Philadelphia: Elsevier; 2015. Fig. 10.9.)

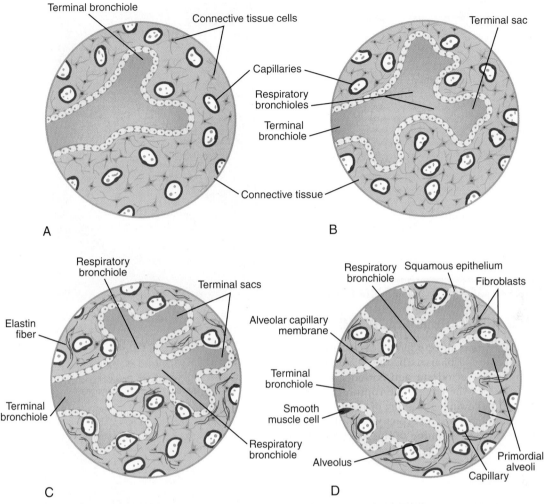

Fig. 9.13   Diagrams of the stages of lung development. (A) Pseudoglandular period (5–17 weeks); (B) canalicular period (16–25 weeks); (C) terminal saccular period (24 weeks–late fetal period); (D) alveolar period (late fetal period–8 years). (Modified from Moore KL, Persaud TVN, & Torchia, MG. *The Developing Human: Clinically Oriented Embryology.* 10th ed. Philadelphia: Elsevier; 2015. Fig. 10.10A–D.)

generations of airways are partially present, including respiratory ducts. Type II pneumocytes begin to appear.

- Canalicular (16–25 weeks)—expansion of the lumina of bronchi and terminal bronchioles and increasing lung vascularity through invasion by capillaries; respiratory bronchioles have formed and divided by primary septa into three to six alveolar ducts with some primordial alveoli (alveolar sacculi). Type I pneumocytes begin to develop from the type II pneumocytes.
- Saccular (24 weeks–late fetal period)—the saccules are lined with type I and II pneumocytes. The septa contain a double layer of capillaries. The capillaries and primordial alveoli form a blood–air barrier (type I pneumocyte, basal membrane, capillary endothelium) across which gas exchange could occur. Type II pneumocytes begin to secrete increasing amounts of surfactant.
- Alveolar stage (34 weeks–8 years)—small protrusions develop, grow and further subdivide along the primary septa forming the alveoli. Each alveoli is delineated by a secondary septum. Approximately 95% of mature alveoli develop postnatally and most are formed by 3 years of age, although it is thought that new alveoli are added until approximately 8 years of age.

The transition from dependence on the placenta for gas exchange to autonomous gas exchange requires the production of sufficient surfactant in the alveolar sacs, the maturation of lung structure to support gas exchange, and the establishment of parallel pulmonary and systemic circulations.

DEVELOPMENT OF THE LARYNX

The epithelium of the larynx develops from endoderm of the cranial portion of the laryngotracheal tube, while the cartilages develop from the mesenchyme (derived from neural crest cells) in the fourth and sixth pharyngeal arches. Mesenchymal proliferation also produces arytenoid swellings which grow toward the tongue, converting the slit-like aperture of the laryngotracheal tube into a T-shaped laryngeal inlet (Fig. 9.14). Rapid proliferation of the laryngeal epithelium results in temporary occlusion of the laryngeal lumen. During recanalisation (by about week 10) the laryngeal ventricles, vocal folds and vestibular folds are formed. The fourth and sixth arches also contribute myoblasts toward the formation of laryngeal muscles, which are innervated by the laryngeal branches of the vagus nerve that supply these two arches.

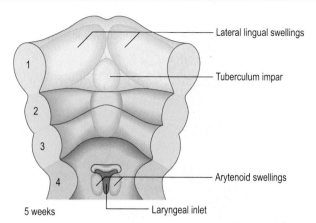

Fig. 9.14 Horizontal section of the embryo at 6 weeks. (Modified from Mitchell B, Sharma R. *Embryology: An Illustrated Colour Text.* 2nd ed. London: Elsevier; 2009. Fig. 11.5B)

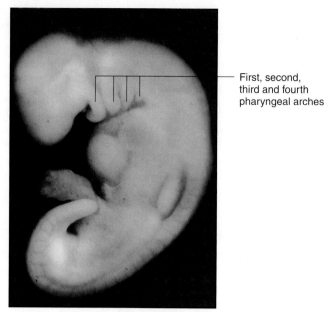

Fig. 9.15 Lateral view of the embryo at 28 days. (Modified from Moore KL, Persaud TVN, & Torchia, MG. *The Developing Human: Clinically Oriented Embryology.* 10th ed. Philadelphia: Elsevier; 2015. Fig. 5.9A, B)

DEVELOPMENT OF THE HEAD AND NECK

FORMATION OF THE MOUTH (STOMODEUM)

The stomodeum begins as an ectodermal depression, separated from the primordial pharynx by the bilaminar) oropharyngeal membrane (ectoderm and endoderm layers). Late in the fourth week the membrane ruptures, opening the stomodeum and allowing continuity of the developing respiratory and alimentary systems (pharynx) with the amniotic cavity. The ectodermal lining of the first pharyngeal arch (see below) forms the oral epithelium.

PHARYNGEAL ARCHES

In week 4, neural crest cells migrate into the developing head and neck regions resulting in the formation of four pairs of pharyngeal arches that are visible on the surface of the embryo (arches 5 and 6 are rudimentary), each separated by a pharyngeal groove (Fig. 9.15). The arches are covered with ectoderm, lined with endoderm and have a mesenchymal core; the latter is derived from proliferating neural crest cells (Fig. 9.16). Concurrently, paraxial myogenic mesodermal cells migrate into the arches, providing muscle primordia. Endothelial cells and angioblasts from the lateral mesoderm also invade the arches. Each pharyngeal arch is comprised of the following: an artery arising from the truncus arteriosus of the primordial heart and exiting at the dorsal aorta; a rod of cartilage; muscles; and motor and sensory nerves (from the neuroectoderm.) As growth occurs, the first arch is separated into maxillary and mandibular prominences (Fig. 9.17). By the end of week 5 the second arch overgrows the third and fourth arches, forming the cervical sinus which disappears 2 weeks later, giving the neck a smooth contour (see Video 9.3).

ARCH DERIVATIVES

FIRST ARCH

- Cartilage (Meckel's cartilage)
  - Proximodorsal – malleus, incus, anterior ligament of malleus, sphenomandibular ligament
  - Ventral – primordium of mandible

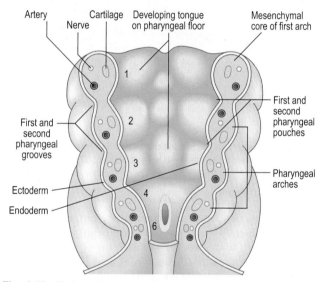

Fig. 9.16 Horizontal section of the cranial region of the embryo at approximately 28 days. (Adapted from Mitchell B, Sharma R. *Embryology: An Illustrated Colour Text.* 2nd ed. London: Elsevier; 2009. Fig. 11.2.)

- Muscle
  - Temporalis, masseter, pterygoids, mylohyoid, digastic (anterior belly), tensor tympani, tensor veli palatini
- Nerve
  - Trigeminal (CN V)
- Artery
  - Portions of the maxillary and external carotid arteries.

SECOND ARCH (REICHERT CARTILAGE)

- Cartilage
  - Styloid process, portion of the stapes, stylohyoid ligament, lesser cornu of the hyoid

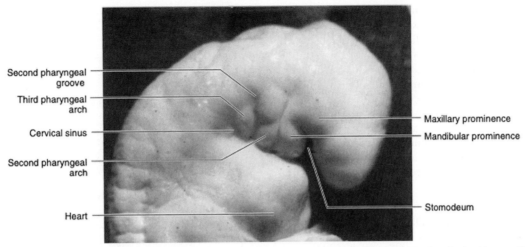

Fig. 9.17 Micrograph of the 32-day-old embryo. (Modified from Moore KL, Persaud TVN, & Torchia, MG. *The Developing Human: Clinically Oriented Embryology.* 10th ed. Philadelphia: Elsevier; 2015. Fig. 5.12A.)

- Muscle
  - Buccinator, auricularis, frontalis, platysma, orbicularis oris and oculi, stapedius, stylohyoid, digastric (posterior belly)
- Nerve
  - Facial (CN VII)
- Artery
  - Stems of the stapedial arteries.

THIRD ARCH

- Cartilage
  - Greater cornu of the hyoid bone, superior cornu of the thyroid cartilage
- Muscle
  - Stylopharyngeus
- Nerve
  - Glossopharyngeal (CN IX)
- Artery
  - Common carotid artery, internal carotid arteries.

FOURTH ARCH (AND COMPONENTS OF THE RUDIMENTARY SIXTH ARCH)

- Cartilage
  - laryngeal cartilages (except for the epiglottis)
- Muscle
  - cricothyroid, levator veli palatini, constrictors of pharynx, intrinsic muscles of the larynx, oesophageal striated muscle
- Nerve
  - Recurrent laryngeal and superior laryngeal branches of vagus (CN X)
- Artery
  - Portion of the aortic arch, proximal right subclavian
  - Proximal left and right pulmonary artery, ductus arteriosus.

PHARYNGEAL GROOVES AND MEMBRANES

The first pair of grooves forms the external acoustic meatus while the first membrane contributes to the tympanic membrane. The other grooves and membranes degenerate.

PHARYNGEAL POUCHES

The endodermal lining of the pharynx develops four pairs of internal pouches (Fig. 9.16), in alignment with the external pharyngeal grooves – the pouch endoderm and groove ectoderm contact each other to form double layered pharyngeal membranes.

PHARYNGEAL POUCH DERIVATIVES

- First pouch
  - Tympanic cavity, mastoid antrum, pharyngotympanic tube
- Second pouch
  - Tonsillar fossa, tonsillar crypts
- Third pouch
  - Inferior parathyroid gland, thymus
- Fourth pouch
  - Superior parathyroid gland.

FORMATION OF THE THYROID GLAND

Early in week 4, a small bud, the thyroid primordium, develops from the medial floor (endoderm) of the embryonic pharynx (Fig. 9.18) and combines with tissue from the two

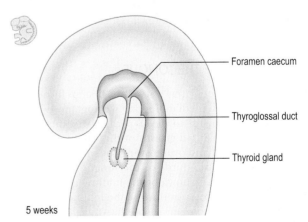

Fig. 9.18 Sagittal image of the embryo at approximately 5 weeks. (Modified from Mitchell B, Sharma R. *Embryology: An Illustrated Colour Text.* 2nd ed. London: Elsevier; 2009. Fig. 11.6B.)

lateral fourth pharyngeal pouches. The median components form the follicular cells, whereas the lateral pouch components provide the parafollicular cells (C cells). With growth of the embryo and the thyroid primordium, the developing thyroid changes its relative position in the neck, passing ventral to the developing hyoid bone and laryngeal cartilages. Connectivity with the tongue is maintained briefly by the thyroglossal duct. At 7 weeks, the thyroid primordium has divided into right and left lobes, connected by the isthmus, and it has assumed its normal location in the neck. The thyroglossal duct normally degenerates and a pit (the foramen cecum in the tongue dorsum) persists as a remnant.

HISTOGENESIS OF THE THYROID AND PARATHYROID GLANDS

THYROID

The initial solid endodermal tissue of the thyroid gland is invaded by surrounding blood vessels and mesenchyme, and it disaggregates into a network of epithelial cords. The cords further divide into small cellular clusters, developing a lumen, with the follicular cells arranged as a single layer surrounding the thyroid follicles. Thyrocytes differentiate from the follicle cells and begin to produce triiodothyronine (T3) and thyroxine (T4). Colloid in the follicles is identifiable by about week 11 and acts as a reservoir for thyroid hormones. Thyroid hormone is required for normal fetal brain development and as early as the first trimester, before the fetal thyroid gland is functioning. Only by 20 weeks are sufficient levels of thyroid-stimulating hormone (TSH) produced by the fetal pituitary and thyroxine levels increase, reaching adult levels at 35 weeks. Before these systems mature, maternal thyroid hormone is provided via the placenta, whereas TSH is produced by the placenta and fetal pancreas. The hormone calcitonin is produced by the C (parafollicular) cells within the thyroid.

PARATHYROID GLANDS

Similar to the thyroid gland, the endoderm of the dorsal third and fourth pouches proliferates, forming small cellular nodules. Blood vessels and mesenchyme invade the nodules to form capillary networks within the glands. Although the predominant chief cells that produce parathyroid hormone become active in the fetus, the large clusters of oxyphil cells do not form until puberty, and their role is unclear.

DEVELOPMENT OF THE TONGUE

Near the end of week 4, as a result of first arch mesenchymal proliferation, a median lingual swelling and two lateral lingual swellings begin to develop rostral to the foramen cecum (Fig. 9.19). Rapid growth of the lateral swellings results in their fusion and overgrowing the medial swelling, to form the anterior two-thirds of the tongue (oral tongue). The plane of fusion is shown by the midline groove and lingual septum. The posterior third of the tongue (pharyngeal tongue) develops from the hypopharyngeal eminence, a swelling of tissue from the ventromedial third and fourth pharyngeal arches (Fig. 9.19). Although a similar more anterior swelling, the copula, develops from the second arch-

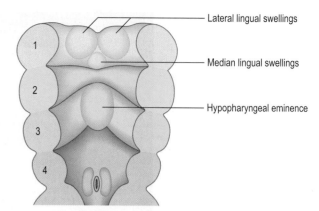

Fig. 9.19 Horizontal sections through the embryo pharynx. (Modified from Mitchell B, Sharma R. *Embryology: An Illustrated Colour Text.* 2nd ed. London: Elsevier; 2009. Fig. 11.5A.)

es, it is overgrown by the hypopharyngeal eminence. The terminal sulcus is the approximate demarcation between the oral and pharyngeal parts of the tongue. The epiglottis develops from the caudal part of the hypopharyngeal eminence. Muscles of the tongue develop from the second to fifth occipital myotomes. The hypoglossal nerve is brought along with the developing muscle and innervates all of the muscles except the palatoglossus, which is supplied by fibres arising from the vagus nerve. The sensory supply to most of the tongue mucosa is the lingual branch of the mandibular division of the trigeminal nerve (first arch nerve). The vallate and foliate papillae appear at approximately week 10, close to terminal branches of the glossopharyngeal nerve, and before the fungiform papillae form near terminations of the chorda tympani branch of the facial nerve. Development of the taste buds within the papillae follows thereafter due, in part, to invading gustatory nerve cells. The pharyngeal tongue is innervated mainly by the third arch glossopharyngeal nerve although a small portion anterior to the epiglottis is innervated by the fourth arch, vagus nerve.

DEVELOPMENT OF THE FACE

Active growth of the cranial mesenchyme results in the formation of the following areas that contribute to the development of the face during weeks 4 to 8: frontonasal prominence, lateral and medial nasal prominences and the maxillary and mandibular prominences. The maxillary and mandibular prominences, derivatives of the first pair of pharyngeal arches, form the lateral and caudal boundaries of the stomodeum, whereas the frontonasal prominence forms the rostral boundary (Fig. 9.20A). By about day 28, nasal placodes develop from surface ectoderm within the inferolateral parts of the frontonasal prominence. Mesenchyme on the margins of the placodes proliferates to form the C-shaped medial and lateral nasal prominences (Fig. 9.20B). The nasal placodes then become sunken nasal pits, and later form the nares and nasal cavities. The maxillary prominences grow medially towards, and then fuse with, the nasal prominences, pushing the latter toward the median plane of the face. Merging of the medial nasal and maxillary prominences results in continuity of the upper jaw and lip and separation of the nasal pits from the stomodeum (Fig. 9.20C). The cleft between the maxillary and lateral

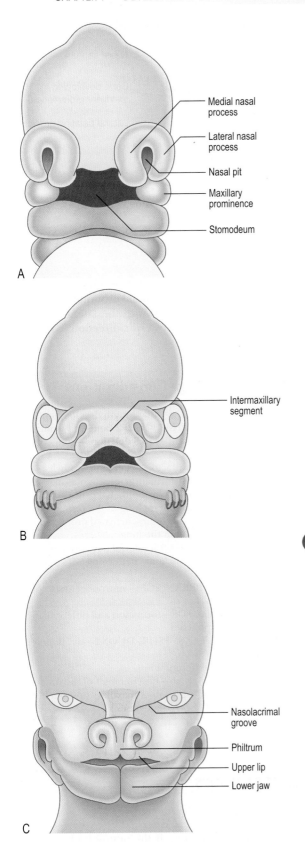

Fig. 9.20 Diagram showing the major components of face development at approximately (A) 6 weeks, (B) 7 weeks and (C) 8 weeks. (From Mitchell B, Sharma R. *Embryology: An Illustrated Colour Text.* 2nd ed. London: Elsevier; 2009. Fig. 11.7B–D)

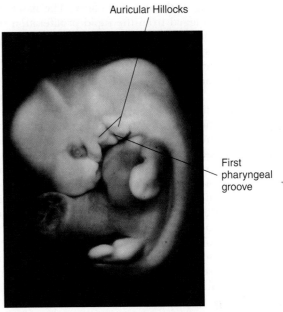

Fig. 9.21 Lateral view of the embryo at approximately 42 days. (Modified from Moore KL, Persaud TVN, & Torchia, MG. *The Developing Human: Clinically Oriented Embryology.* 10th ed. Philadelphia: Elsevier; 2015. Fig. 5.14A, B)

nasal prominence becomes the nasolacrimal groove, later forming the nasolacrimal duct with the expanded superior end forming the lacrimal sac (Fig. 9.20C). The nasolacrimal duct only becomes completely patent in infancy. The medial nasal prominences merge and form the intermaxillary segment, the precursor of the philtrum, premaxillary part of the maxilla and associated gingiva, and the primary palate. The upper lip is formed entirely from the fusion of the maxillary prominences (see Video 9.4).

During the fetal period, facial growth continues at a slower pace, and the relative positions and proportions of the face are further defined. For instance, as the brain enlarges, the cranial cavity expands resulting in the orbits moving to a forward-facing orientation.

EXTERNAL EARS

By about day 35, six auricular hillocks form from mesenchyme and adjacent to the first pharyngeal groove (Fig. 9.21) The hillocks represent the early auricle whereas the pharyngeal groove will form the external acoustic meatus. Although early in development the auricles are located low in the developing neck, the expansion of the mandibles and relative growth of the head and face result in the auricles being repositioned at the level of the eyes.

DEVELOPMENT OF NASAL CAVITIES AND PARANASAL SINUSES

Nasal placodes continue to invaginate, forming nasal pits and, in turn, primordial nasal sacs. The sacs grow in a dorsal direction, ventral to the developing forebrain. Although the sacs are initially separated from the oral cavity by the oronasal membrane, by week 7 the membrane undergoes apoptosis resulting in the initial choanae. The nasal cavity soon becomes plugged from the rapid proliferation of its epithelial cells, but by week 17 a lumen is formed by apoptosis. During this remodelling, the superior, middle and inferior nasal conchae develop from the lateral walls of the nasal cavities. The epithelium in the roof of each nasal cavity differentiates into olfactory epithelium with some cells further differentiating into specialised neurons—olfactory receptor cells; the associated axons constitute the olfactory nerves with connection to the olfactory bulbs of the brain.

Only the maxillary sinuses begin to form in the prenatal period and are poorly developed at birth. Initially, the maxillary and ethmoid sinuses form from diverticula of the walls of the nasal cavities and later become pneumatic extensions of the nasal cavities in the adjacent bones. The diverticular openings form the orifices of the nasal sinuses. Anterior and posterior components develop from the ethmoid sinuses and contribute to the formation of the frontal sinuses and sphenoidal sinuses, respectively, at approximately 2 years of age. All of the sinuses begin to grow more rapidly in later childhood. The maxillary sinuses are not fully developed until all the permanent teeth have erupted. Growth of the paranasal sinuses alters the size and shape of the face and changes the resonance of the voice during adolescence.

DEVELOPMENT OF THE PALATE

In week 6, merging of the internal surfaces of the medial nasal prominences results in the formation of the mesenchymal-derived primary palate. The primary palate undergoes ossification and becomes the premaxillary part of the maxilla and a small portion of the definitive palate anterior to the incisive fossa. The secondary palate develops from lateral palatine processes projecting from the internal surface of the maxillary prominences and inferomedially on each side of the tongue (Fig. 9.22). By week 9, facilitated by the production of hyaluronic acid in the mesenchyme, the lateral palatine processes assume a horizontal position above the tongue. The tissue of the anterior secondary palate also undergoes ossification to form the hard palate, whereas the posterior portions fuse and remain as soft tissue, forming the soft palate and uvula. Visible in young adults, an irregular suture is seen from the incisive fossa to the alveolar process of the maxilla (between the lateral incisors and cuspids) which indicates where the primary and secondary palates fused.

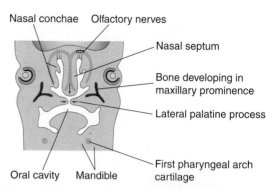

Fig. 9.23 Sagittal section of the developing head. (Modified from Moore KL, Persaud TVN, & Torchia, MG. *The Developing Human: Clinically Oriented Embryology.* 10th ed. Philadelphia: Elsevier; 2015. Fig. 9.36E.)

The tissue for the nasal septum originates from inferior growth of the merged median nasal prominences (Fig. 9.23). The primordial septum fuses with the lateral palatine processes, in an anterior to posterior direction, completed by the end of week 11.

Molecular Biology Considerations

- Candidate genes on 15q—diaphragm development
- GATA6, GATA4, ZFPM2, NR2F2 and WT1 mutations (15q26) and 8p23.1 and 4p16.3 deletions—congenital diaphragmatic hernia
- Thyroid transcription factor 1, hepatocyte nuclear factor 3β and GATA6—transformation of endodermal foregut cells to form respiratory-type epithelial cells
- FGF10—formation and branching of the respiratory buds
- SOX17, Wnt7b signaling—mesenchymal proliferation and blood vessel formation in the lung
- Hox genes expression—craniofacial development
- Shh, Dlx2—formation and patterning of pharyngeal arches
- BMP, PRRX1, PRRX, FGFs—morphogenesis of the mandible
- Retinoic acid, Wnt, FGF—formation and differentiation of the pharyngeal pouches
- TITF1, FOXE1, PAX8, TSHR, DUOX2—development of the thyroid
- MASH1—C-cell differentiation
- PAX3, PAX7, Dlx5, Dlx6—development of the tongue
- PDGFRA signaling—growth of maxillary prominences
- WNT and PRICKLE1—palatogenesis

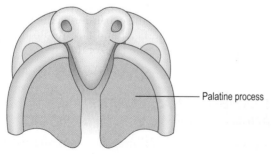

Fig. 9.22 Diagrammatic section of the roof of the mouth at week 6. (Modified from Mitchell B, Sharma R. *Embryology: An Illustrated Colour Text.* 2nd ed. London: Elsevier; 2009. Fig. 11.9B.)

CLINICAL ISSUES

GASTROSCHISIS

During embryonic folding, if the lateral body folds do not fuse completely, a defect in the abdominal wall occurs resulting in protrusion of the abdominal viscera. The exact cause for this lack of fusion has not been identified. Gastroschisis is usually found to the right of the umbilical cord rather than in the midline. In utero, the herniated bowel is uncovered and floating in the amniotic fluid. Depending on the size of the defect, the stomach and liver may also protrude. Treatment may be accomplished through primary surgical closure (about 60% of cases) or, if the viscera do not easily fit back into the abdomen, the bowel can be protected outside the abdomen (in a polymer pouch) allowing the viscera to be reduced into the abdominal cavity over days, followed by repair of the abdominal wall defect.

CONGENITAL DIAPHRAGMATIC HERNIA

In congenital diaphragmatic hernia (CDH), a defect in the formation of the diaphragm, most commonly on the left posterolateral side, may lead to herniation of abdominal contents into the thoracic cavity, interference with anatomic lung development, delay of physiological maturation of the lungs and inhibition of postpartum lung inflation. CDH typically is a result of defective formation or fusion of the pleuroperitoneal membranes with the remaining embryonic components of the diaphragm. If this fusion is not completed before the physiological intestinal hernia is reduced, at week 10, intestinal viscera may pass into the thorax, pushing the lungs and heart anteriorly and compressing the lungs. Lung hypoplasia results from the lack of space for normal development. For the neonate, pulmonary hypertension because of decreased vascular cross-sectional area and pulmonary vasoconstriction also contribute to the morbidity of CDH. Surgical reduction of the hernia and repair of the diaphragmatic defect may cause the lungs to become aerated and achieve their normal size. Enhanced ventilatory support and extracorporeal membrane oxygenation have improved the outcomes from CDH, although overall mortality rates are approximately 50%.

CHAOS

Congenital high airway obstruction syndrome (CHAOS) is caused by atresia, stenosis or a web-like blockage of the trachea or larynx from defective recanalisation. Fetuses with CHAOS syndrome may have dilated airways, overdistended lungs and a flattened or everted diaphragm; fetal hydrops may also develop. Ex utero intrapartum treatment of the fetus may be required to provide oxygenation through a tracheostomy or other procedure.

TRACHEOESOPHAGEAL FISTULA

Lack of complete separation of the foregut into oesophageal and respiratory components from incomplete fusion of the tracheoesophageal folds results in a tracheoesophageal fistula (TEF), the most common defect of the lower respiratory tract. The most frequent variant of TEF involves the superior oesophagus, with the inferior portion of the oesophagus joining the trachea near its bifurcation. Because swallowing is not possible in this situation, polyhydramnios frequently occurs.

RESPIRATORY DISTRESS SYNDROME

A deficiency of pulmonary surfactant results in lungs that are underinflated and alveoli which contain a proteinaceous fluid thought to be derived partially from injured pulmonary epithelium. Factors that contribute to surfactant deficiency include: fetal immaturity, prolonged intrauterine asphyxia that damages type II alveolar cells, sepsis, aspiration and pneumonia. Maternal antenatal treatment with glucocorticoid accelerates fetal lung development and surfactant production. Neonatal administration of exogenous surfactant is also utilised to improve outcomes.

BRONCHOGENIC CYSTS

Dilation of the terminal bronchi can occur from a disturbances in normal bronchial development resulting in pouch-like formations filled with fluid, air or both. Compressive symptoms (e.g., dysphagia), infection and malignant transformation can occur.

LUNG HYPOPLASIA

Lung growth is restricted in fetuses with CDH owing to compression by abdominal viscera. Beyond significantly reduced lung volume, hypertrophy of smooth muscle in the pulmonary arteries occurs leading to pulmonary hypertension, reduced pulmonary blood flow and shunting of blood through the ductus arteriosus; this pulmonary insufficiency is the primary cause of fatalities from CDH.

THYROGLOSSAL DUCT CYST

Cysts may form along the former thyroglossal duct if the duct does not undergo involution. These cysts are most commonly located in the tongue or anterior neck just inferior to the hyoid bone. The cysts are typically asymptomatic and may contain some thyroid tissue.

FIRST ARCH SYNDROMES

Abnormal development of components of the first arch, likely because of insufficient migration of neural crest cells, results in defects of the eyes, ears, mandible and palate, which together constitute a first arch syndrome. There are two main first arch disorders:

- Treacher Collins syndrome (mandibulofacial dysostosis)—autosomal-dominant disorder with malar hypoplasia, down-slanting palpebral fissures, defects of the lower eyelids, and abnormalities of the external ears and sometimes of the middle and inner ears.
- Pierre Robin sequence—typically occurs de novo and is characterised by micrognathia, glossoptosis, cleft palate, airway obstruction and defects of the eyes and ears.

CLEFT PALATE AND LIP

Palate clefts arise from failure of the lateral palatine process to fuse with:

- the primary palate (anterior cleft)
- each other and the nasal septum (posterior cleft)
- the primary palate, with each other, and the nasal septum (secondary palate cleft).

Some clefts appear as part of single mutant gene or chromosomal syndromes or effects of teratogenic substances.

These defects are usually classified into two major groups according to developmental criteria, with the incisive fossa used as a reference landmark:

- Anterior cleft defects—cleft lip with or without a cleft of the alveolar part of the maxilla. A complete anterior cleft extends through the upper lip and alveolar part of the maxilla to the incisive fossa, separating the anterior and posterior parts of the palate.
- Posterior cleft defects—clefts of the secondary palate that extend through the soft and hard regions of the palate to the incisive fossa, separating the anterior and posterior parts of the palate.

The lip clefts may be:

- unilateral—failure of one side of the maxillary prominence to unite with the merged medial nasal prominence. A tissue bridge (Simonart band) sometimes joins the parts of the incomplete cleft lip.
- bilateral—failure of both maxillary prominences to meet and unite with the merged medial nasal prominences. Significant deformation occurs because of the loss of continuity, which affects function of the orbicularis oris muscle that normally closes the mouth and purses the lips.

Case Outcome

Physical examination was normal except for the left submandibular mass. Blood work was normal except for a mild leucocytosis. Ultrasound examination demonstrated an echogenic, homogenous cystic mass measuring 3.1 cm × 3.6 cm. Three weeks later, magnetic resonance imaging was performed as the mass had not decreased in size. The imaging demonstrated a 3.0-cm × 3.4-cm mass, anterior to the sternocleidomastoid muscle, with enhancing tissue toward the left tonsillar fossa, consistent with a second branchial cleft cyst. HD was referral to an otolaryngologist.

Additional reflection: What specific embryological process led to the formation of this cyst? What significance is the extension of enhancement toward the tonsillar fossa? What role does watchful waiting play in the follow-up to HD and what are the risks associated with not treating this branchial cyst? What role does surgery play and under what conditions might it be considered?

QUESTIONS

1. Laryngeal cartilages are derived mainly from:
   a. second and third pharyngeal arches
   b. third and fourth pharyngeal arches
   c. third, fourth and fifth pharyngeal arches
   d. fourth and sixth pharyngeal arches
   e. fourth and fifth pharyngeal arches

2. If the palatine processes fail to fuse together and also fuse with the nasal cartilage, the anomaly that results would be a cleft of the:
   a. uvula
   b. primary palate
   c. secondary palate
   d. primary and secondary palates
   e. medial nasal prominences

3. Pulmonary surfactant is produced by type II alveolar epithelial cells, beginning at approximately how many weeks?
   a. 16
   b. 20
   c. 24
   d. 28
   e. 32

4. Lung hypoplasia is commonly associated with which one of the following?
   a. Congenital diaphragmatic hernia
   b. CHAOS
   c. Tracheoesophageal fistula
   d. Respiratory distress syndrome
   e. First arch syndromes

5. The septum transversum initially separates the developing:
   a. heart and lungs
   b. oesophagus and trachea
   c. left and right lungs
   d. heart and liver
   e. lungs and colon.

BIBLIOGRAPHY

Clifton MS, Wylkan ML. Congenital diaphragmatic hernia and diaphragmatic eventration. Clin Perinatol 2017;44:773–9.

Logan SM, Ruest L-B, Benson MD, Svoboda KHH. Extracellular matrix in secondary palate development. Anat Rec 2019; https://doi.org/10.1002/ar.24263.

Nilsson M, Fagman H. Development of the thyroid. Development 2017;144:2123–40.

Parada C, Han D, Chai Y. Molecular and cellular regulatory mechanisms of tongue myogenesis. J Dent Res 2012;91:528–35.

Pu Q, Patel K, Huang R. The lateral plate mesoderm: a novel source of skeletal muscle. Results Probl Cell Differ 2017;56:142–63.

Sefton EM, Galardi M, Kardon G. Developmental origin and morphogenesis of the diaphragm, an essential mammalian muscle. Dev Biol 2018;440:64–73.

Som PM, Grapin-Botton A. The current embryology of the foregut and its derivatives. Neurographics 2016;6:43–63.

Spinelli C, Rosi L, Strambi S, et al. Branchial cleft and pouch anomalies in childhood: a report of 50 surgical cases. J Endocrinol Invest 2016;39:529–35.

Development of the Nervous System, Eyes and Ears

Case Scenario

JJ is a 22-year-old pregnant woman who developed rubella during her 10th week of gestation. Baby male EJ was born at 38 weeks of gestation with a birth weight of 3250 g. Physical examination of the infant was normal. His automatic auditory brainstem response was also normal. No congenital cardiac anomaly was detected on echocardiography.

Questions for reflection: How would JJ have developed a rubella infection during pregnancy? Could this have resulted from a rubella inoculation? Given the history, what specific physical abnormalities might have been suspected, if any could have existed in EJ? Would there be are any blood tests that might be informative and why? What does a normal auditory brainstem response test indicate?

DEVELOPMENT OF THE NERVOUS SYSTEM

During week 4, the notochord and paraxial mesenchyme induce the overlying ectoderm to differentiate into the neural plate and later the neural groove, folds, crest and tube. Cranial to the fourth pair of somites, the neural plate and tube represent the developing brain, while caudally, they represent the future spinal cord. The neural crest contributes cells that form most of the peripheral and autonomic nervous system. Fusion of the neural folds to form the neural tube begins at the fifth somite and proceeds at multiple locations until the rostral and caudal neuropores close at approximately day 25 and 27, respectively, which coincides with the development of neural tube vascularisation. The neural canal forms the brain ventricles and the central canal of the spinal cord (see Video 10.1).

As development of the primordial nervous system continues, the neural tube thickens with the growth of pseudostratified, columnar neuroepithelium that forms the ventricular zone (Fig. 10.2). A neuroepithelial marginal zone develops into white matter as nerve cell body axons extend into it from the brain, spinal cord and ganglia. Neuroblasts from the ventricular zone migrate to form the intermediate zone and differentiate into neurons. Glioblasts also differentiate from neuroepithelial cells and migrate from the ventricular zone into the intermediate and marginal zones to eventually form astrocytes and oligodendrocytes. Following formation of neuroblasts and glioblasts, the neuroepithelium differentiates into ependymal cells. Microglia invade the developing brain and spine from the bone marrow following vascularisation of the nervous system.

DEVELOPMENT OF THE BRAIN

As the cranial neural folds undergo fusion and the rostral neuropore closes, three primary brain vesicles develop: prosencephalon (forebrain), mesencephalon (midbrain) and the rhombencephalon (hindbrain). Further division of the prosencephalon produces the telencephalon and the diencephalon (Fig. 10.3). Rapid and differential growth within the developing brain produces the midbrain, pontine and cervical flexures, resulting in considerable variation in wall thickness and in the position of the grey and white matter. The pontine flexure further divides the rhombencephalon into the metencephalon and myelencephalon, while the cervical flexure separates the myelencephalon from the spinal cord. The sulcus limitans extends cranially to the midbrain/forebrain junction, with the alar and basal plates seen only in the midbrain and hindbrain.

RHOMBENCEPHALON

The myelencephalon becomes the medulla oblongata, and the metencephalon becomes the pons and cerebellum. The neural canal of the rhombencephalon becomes the fourth ventricle and the central canal in the medulla. Given its developmental proximity, the caudal portion of the medulla resembles the spinal cord developmentally and structurally. However, unlike neuroblasts of the spinal cord, those from the myelencephalon alar plates migrate into the marginal zone to form the gracile and cuneate nuclei, which are associated with gracile and cuneate nerve tracts that enter the medulla from the spinal cord (Fig. 10.4). Corticospinal fibre bundles (pyramids) develop in the ventral medulla from fibres descending from the developing cerebral cortex. The pontine flexure results in the lateral walls of the medulla moving laterally, with its roof plate thinned and the alar plates being repositioned to be lateral to the basal plates such that the motor nuclei develop medial to the sensory nuclei. Medullar basal plate neuroblasts develop into motor neurons and form nuclei in three bilateral cell columns: general somatic efferent, special visceral efferent and general visceral efferent. Medullar alar plate neuroblasts form nuclei in four bilateral columns: general visceral afferent, special visceral afferent, general somatic afferent and special somatic afferent (Fig. 10.5).

The metencephalon forms the pons and cerebellum, and the cavity of the metencephalon forms the superior part of the fourth ventricle (Fig. 10.6). Creation of the pontine flexure results in separation of the lateral walls of the pons and spreading of the grey matter in the floor of the fourth ventricle. Neuroblasts in the basal plates develop into motor

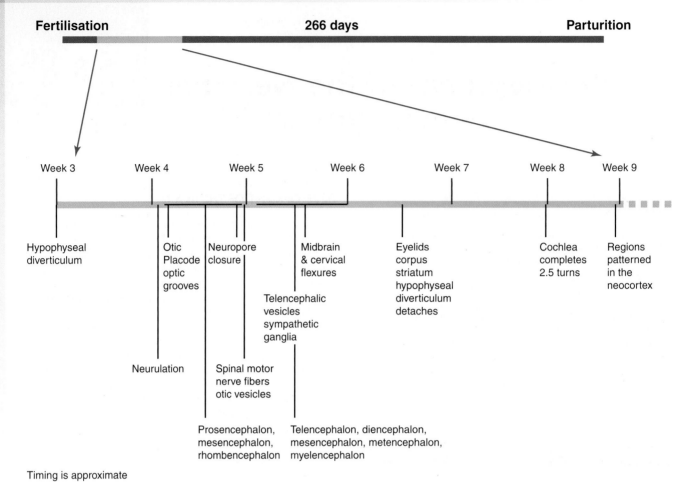

Timing is approximate

Fig. 10.1   Timeline of development related to the nervous system, eyes and ears.

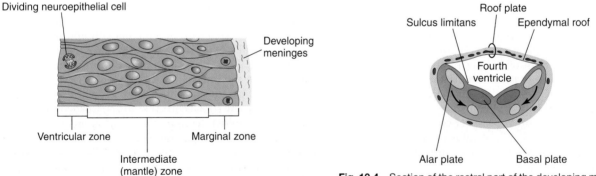

Fig. 10.2   Section of the wall of the developing neural tube. (Modified from Moore KL, Persaud TVN, Torchia MG. *The Developing Human: Clinically Oriented Embryology.* 10th ed. Philadelphia: Elsevier; 2015.)

Fig. 10.4   Section of the rostral part of the developing medulla. (Modified from Moore KL, Persaud TVN, Torchia MG. *The Developing Human: Clinically Oriented Embryology.* 10th ed. Philadelphia: Elsevier; 2015.)

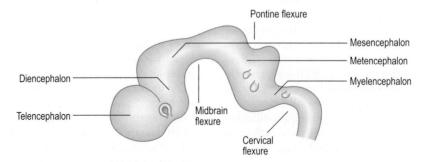

Fig. 10.3   Lateral view of the developing central nervous system of a 6-week embryo. (Modified from Mitchell B, Sharma R. *Embryology: An Illustrated Colour Text.* 2nd ed. London: Elsevier; 2009.)

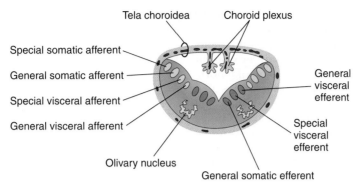

Fig. 10.5 Section of the rostral part of the developing medulla showing further differentiation of the afferent and efferent columns. (Modified from Moore KL, Persaud TVN, Torchia MG. *The Developing Human: Clinically Oriented Embryology.* 10th ed. Philadelphia: Elsevier; 2015.)

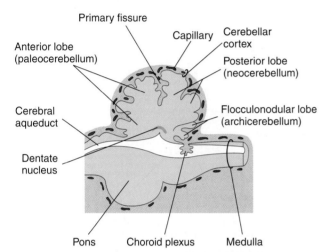

Fig. 10.6 Transverse section of the developing pons and cerebellum. (Modified from Moore KL, Persaud TVN, Torchia MG. *The Developing Human: Clinically Oriented Embryology.* 10th ed. Philadelphia: Elsevier; 2015.)

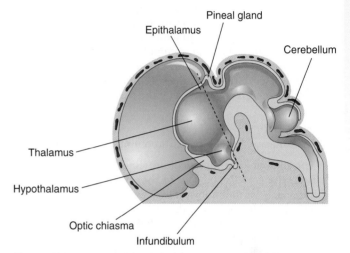

Fig. 10.7 Median section of the brain at 8 weeks. (Modified from Moore KL, Persaud TVN, Torchia MG. *The Developing Human: Clinically Oriented Embryology.* 10th ed. Philadelphia: Elsevier; 2015.)

nuclei. As the dorsal parts of the alar plates thicken, they form cerebellar swellings and project into the fourth ventricle. With further growth, the two swellings fuse, overgrow that portion of the fourth ventricle, and overlap the medulla and pons. Cells from the alar plates also form the central nuclei, pontine nuclei, cochlear and vestibular nuclei, and the sensory nuclei of the trigeminal nerve.

MESENCEPHALON

In the mesencephalon, neuroblasts from the alar plates form the superior and inferior colliculi whereas those from the basal plates give rise to red nuclei, nuclei of third and fourth cranial nerves, and reticular nuclei. The corticopontine, corticobulbar and corticospinal fibres grow from the cerebrum and pass through the mesencephalon on their way to the brainstem and spinal cord. The neural canal of the mesencephalon narrows and becomes the cerebral aqueduct.

PROSENCEPHALON

Early in the development of the prosencephalon, two sets of diverticula form: the optic vesicles grow as more cranial lateral outpouchings, and the telencephalic vesicles develop as the primordia of the cerebral hemispheres.

The lateral ventricles form from the cavity of the telencephalon whereas the third ventricle is formed primarily from the cavity of the diencephalon and with a small contribution from the telencephalon.

Bilateral thalami develop from the sides of the third ventricle, bulge in, and in about 70% of cases, fuse in the midline (interthalamic adhesion). The hypothalamus is formed by intermediate zone neuroblasts in the diencephalic walls, with the endocrine and homeostatic controlling nuclei as well as the mammillary bodies developing later. The epithalamus develops from the roof and dorsal portion of the lateral wall of the diencephalons whereas the pineal gland develops from the caudal part of the roof of the diencephalon (Fig. 10.7).

TELENCEPHALON

The lateral diverticula of the telencephalon form the cerebral hemispheres whereas its cavity forms the most anterior portion of the third ventricle. The cerebral hemispheres expand to cover the diencephalon, mesencephalon and rhombencephalon and, in the midline, trap mesenchyme in between which becomes the falx cerebri. The floor of each hemisphere expands and swells to form the corpus striatum while the lateral portions begin to thin, resulting in alterations to the shape of the hemispheres and the lateral ventricles. This reshaping continues as the caudal end of each hemisphere turns ventrally and then rostrally to form the temporal lobe. The thin medial wall of the hemisphere is invaginated along the choroid fissure by vascular pia mater to form the choroid plexus of the temporal horn. As the hemispheres continue to differentiate, fibres that pass through the corpus striatum divide it into caudate and lentiform nuclei, while other fibres (commissures) connect corresponding areas of the cerebral hemispheres with one another including the anterior and hippocampal commissures. The largest cerebral commissure is the corpus callosum, which extends over the roof of the diencephalon in the neonate. The walls of the cerebral hemispheres initially show three zones of the neural tube: ventricular, intermediate and marginal; the subventricular zone appears later. Cells of the intermediate zone migrate into the marginal zone and give rise to the cortical layers. The grey matter is located peripherally, and axons from its cell bodies pass centrally to form the large volume of white matter. The surface of the cerebral hemispheres starts off smooth but rapid growth causes infolding of the cerebral cortex, forming gyri and sulci, and greatly increasing the surface area.

PITUITARY GLAND

The pituitary gland has two components (Fig. 10.8A, B):

- The hypophyseal diverticulum (Rathke pouch), derived from the ectodermal roof of the stomodeum, forms the anterior lobe (adenohypophysis).
- The neurohypophyseal diverticulum, derived from the neuroectoderm of the diencephalon, forms the posterior lobe (neurohypophysis); neuroepithelial cells differentiate into pituicytes, the primary cells of the posterior lobe of the pituitary gland.

CHOROID PLEXUSES AND CEREBROSPINAL FLUID

The ependymal roof of each cerebral hemisphere, third and fourth ventricles, and medial walls of the lateral ventricles, together with the associated highly vascular pia mater, differentiate into the various choroid plexuses. The epithelial lining of the choroid plexus is derived from neuroepithelium, whereas the stroma develops from mesenchymal cells. The choroid plexuses secrete ventricular fluid, which becomes cerebrospinal fluid (CSF) with later additions of constituents from the surfaces of the brain, spinal cord and the pia–arachnoid layer of the meninges. CSF is critical for brain development as it contains, amongst other critical neurogenic factors, signalling morphogens. Three evaginations in the roof of the fourth ventricle form and rupture to create the median and lateral apertures, which provide a path for the CSF to enter the subarachnoid space.

DEVELOPMENT OF THE SPINAL CORD

Caudal to the fourth pair of somites, the lateral walls of the neural tube thicken into the developing spinal cord, to support the thin roof and floor plates. This thickening produces the sulcus limitans separating the alar (dorsal) and basal (ventral) plates (Fig. 10.9). Alar neuron cell bodies form the dorsal grey columns while the basal plate cell bodies form the ventral and lateral grey columns. In transverse sections these columns are the dorsal, ventral and lateral grey horns,

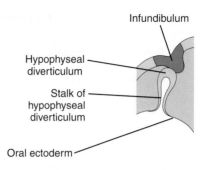

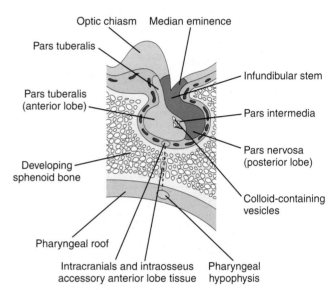

Fig. 10.8 Development of the pituitary gland at (A) approximately 36 days, (B) later fetal period. (Modified from Moore KL, Persaud TVN, Torchia MG. *The Developing Human: Clinically Oriented Embryology.* 10th ed. Philadelphia: Elsevier; 2015.)

respectively. Axons of ventral horn neurons grow out of the spinal cord and form the ventral roots of the spinal nerves. The basal plates continue to enlarge, forming the ventral median fissure.

Dorsal root ganglia cells are derived from neural crest cells and differentiate to have peripheral processes that pass in the spinal nerves to sensory endings in somatic or visceral structures, and central processes that enter the spinal cord as the dorsal roots of spinal nerves.

The spinal cord meninges also develop from neural crest with contributions from mesenchyme. The external layer thickens to form the dura mater while the thin internal layer comprises pia and arachnoid maters (leptomeninges). Contiguous fluid-filled spaces develop within leptomeninges to form the subarachnoid space.

Although early in development, the spinal cord extends the entire length of the vertebral canal and the growth of the vertebral column and dura mater outpaces the cord, resulting in the caudal end of the cord gradually coming to lie at increasingly higher levels: 24-week-old fetus, first sacral vertebra; neonates, second or third lumbar vertebra; adults, inferior border of the first lumbar vertebra. As a result of this shift, the spinal nerve roots run obliquely from the spinal cord to the corresponding level of the vertebral column, especially in the lumbar and sacral regions. Nerve roots inferior

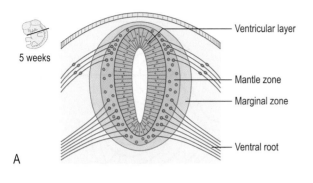

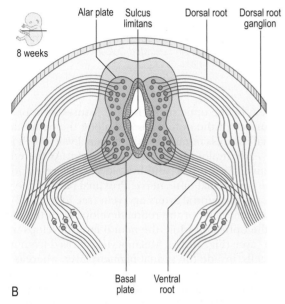

Fig. 10.9 Transverse section of the neural tube at (A) 5 weeks and (B) 8 weeks. (Modified from Moore KL, Persaud TVN, Torchia MG. *The Developing Human: Clinically Oriented Embryology.* 10th ed. Philadelphia: Elsevier; 2015. Fig. 10.2A, B.)

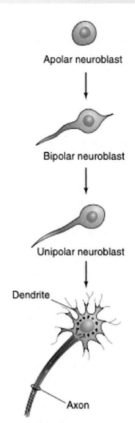

Fig. 10.10 Differentiation of unipolar neuron. (Modified from Moore KL, Persaud TVN, Torchia MG. *The Developing Human: Clinically Oriented Embryology.* 10th ed. Philadelphia: Elsevier; 2015. Fig. 17.9A–D.)

to the medullary cone form the cauda equina. The dura and arachnoid maters, enclosing the subarachnoid space, typically ends at S2 in adults, whereas the pia mater forms the terminal filum which extends from the medullary cone and attaches to the periosteum of the first coccygeal vertebra.

Spinal cord myelination (and function of the fibre tracts) begin in the later fetal period, continuing until about the end of the first postnatal year, with motor roots myelinated before sensory roots.

DEVELOPMENT OF PERIPHERAL NERVOUS SYSTEM

The peripheral nervous system develops primarily from neural crest cells. Almost all peripheral sensory cells begin as bipolar cells. During development, the two processes unite to form unipolar neurons with their peripheral process terminating in a sensory ending and central process entering the spinal cord or brain (Fig. 10.10). Each afferent neuron is closely invested by a satellite cell capsule (derived from neural crest) continuous with the neurilemma. Sensory ganglia of CN V, VII, VIII, IX and X are derived from neural crest cells from the developing brain. Neural crest cells also become neurons of the autonomic ganglia and cells of the chromaffin system.

Motor nerve fibres arise from the spinal cord basal plates, with those fibres associated with each muscle group forming a ventral nerve root. The central processes of the spinal ganglion neuron form bundles that grow into the spinal cord opposite the apex of the dorsal horn of grey matter whereas the distal processes grow towards the ventral nerve root to form a spinal nerve (Fig. 10.9). These mixed spinal nerves have a small dorsal primary ramus, innervating the dorsal axial muscles, vertebrae, posterior intervertebral joints and part of the skin of the back; a larger ventral primary ramus innervates the limbs and ventrolateral parts of the body wall. Limb bud development occurs concurrently with the nerve or the associated spinal cord segment, allowing the nerve fibres to be distributed to the various limb muscles. Peripheral nerve myelin sheaths are formed by the plasma membranes of the neurilemma cells (Schwann cells), derived from neural crest cells. These cells wrap the central and peripheral processes of somatic and visceral sensory neurons, and also around the axons of postsynaptic autonomic motor neurons.

ORIGIN OF THE CRANIAL NERVES

- CN I—cells in the epithelium of the nasal sac
- CN II—neuroblasts in the primordial retina
- CN III—somatic efferent column
- CN IV—somatic efferent column
- CN V—special visceral efferent column
- CN VI—somatic efferent column
- CN VII—special visceral efferent column

- CN VIII—vestibular nerve – semicircular duct cells; cochlear nerve – cochlear duct cells
- CN IX—special visceral efferent column
- CN X—visceral efferent and afferent components
- CN XI—rootlets from the cervical segments of the spinal cord
- CN XII—somatic efferent column.

DEVELOPMENT OF THE AUTONOMIC NERVOUS SYSTEM

In the thoracic region, neural crest cells form preaortic ganglia (e.g., celiac ganglia), terminal ganglia in sympathetic organ plexuses, such as those of the heart, and individual ganglia dorsolateral to the aorta. The latter ganglia become connected by longitudinal nerve fibres to become sympathetic trunks. Later, axons from the lateral horn pass through the ventral root of a spinal nerve and a white ramus communicans to a paravertebral ganglion, to either synapse or to ascend or descend in the sympathetic trunk, synapsing at other levels. Other presynaptic fibres pass through the paravertebral ganglia without synapsing, forming splanchnic nerves to the viscera.

Some presynaptic parasympathetic fibres arise from neurons in nuclei of the brainstem and exit through CN III, VII, IX and X. Other presynaptic parasympathetic fibres arise in the sacral region of the spinal cord. The associated postsynaptic neurons are located in peripheral ganglia or in plexuses near or within the structure being innervated.

DEVELOPMENT OF THE EYES

During formation of the neural tube, the optic grooves evaginate to form diverticula, optic vesicles which, as the brain enlarges, make contact with the surface ectoderm (Fig. 10.11). The proximal stalk of the vesicle narrows to form the optic stalks. The distal end of the optic vesicles expands and induces the surface ectoderm to form lens placodes. The placodes form pits and their edges fuse to form spherical lens vesicles which lose their connection with the surface ectoderm (Fig. 10.12). Simultaneously, the optic vesicles invaginate and form double-walled optic cups that infold around the developing lens. The walls of the optic cups are connected

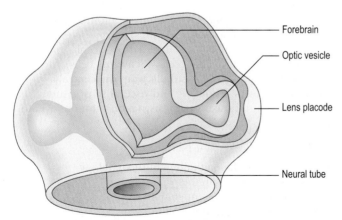

Fig. 10.11 Schematic drawing of embryo forebrain at approximately 28 days. (Modified from Mitchell B, Sharma R. *Embryology: An Illustrated Colour Text.* 2nd ed. London: Elsevier; 2009.)

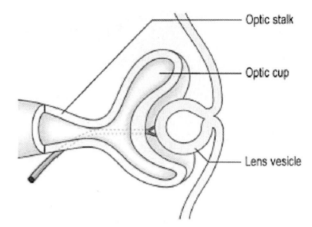

Fig. 10.12 Section of the developing eye. (Modified from Mitchell B, Sharma R. *Embryology: An Illustrated Colour Text.* 2nd ed. London: Elsevier; 2009. Fig. 11.11B.)

to the brain by the optic stalks. Retinal fissures form on the ventral surface of the optic cups and along the optic stalks. The retinal fissures contain vascular mesenchyme which produce the early hyaloid blood artery and vein. As the edges of the retinal fissure fuse, the hyaloid vessels are enclosed within the primordial optic nerve. Proximal parts of the vessels persist as the central artery and vein (see Video 10.2).

The pigment layer of the retina develops from the outer layer of the optic cup while the neural layer develops from the inner layer (Fig. 10.13). Melanocytes, derived from neural crest cells, invade the retinal pigment layer, whereas the developing lens induces proliferation of cells in the neural layer to form a thick neuroepithelium, and subsequently photoreceptors (rods and cones) and the cell bodies of neurons to form the light-sensitive region of the retina, adjacent to the outer retinal pigment epithelium. The intrarenal space disappears later in the fetal period through a relatively weak fusion of the two layers. Axons from ganglion cells in the neural retina grow proximally in the wall of the optic stalk causing the lumen of the optic stalk to be obliterated and the stalk to form the optic nerve. The derivation of the optic stalk means that the optic nerve is surrounded by an outer dural sheath that blends with the sclera, and intermediate thin sheath from arachnoid mater and the inner vascular pia mater sheath. CSF is found in the subarachnoid space between the intermediate and inner sheaths of the optic nerve. Although myelination of the axons begins in the late fetal period, this process is only completed with exposure to light during the first 10-week neonatal period. Neonates are farsighted and can focus only to about 25 cm.

Formation of other components of the eye (Fig. 10.14):

- Pigmented ciliary epithelium is derived from the outer optic cup, whereas the ciliary muscle arises from mesenchyme at the optic cup edge.
- The epithelium of the iris originates from the rim of the optic cup and represents both layers of the optic cup. It is continuous with both layers of the retina. The stroma of the iris is derived from neural crest cells, while its muscles form by transformation of anterior epithelial cells of the iris to smooth muscle cells.
- The lens subcapsular epithelium is derived from the anterior wall of the lens vesicle while the primary lens fibres

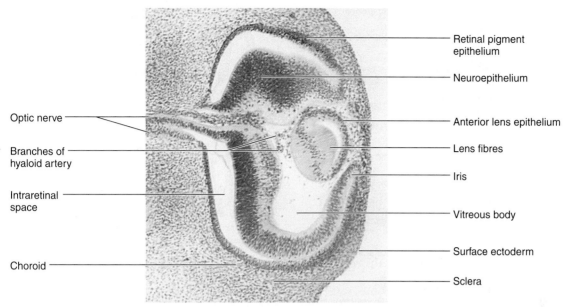

Fig. 10.13 Photomicrograph of a sagittal section of the eye at 44 days. (Modified from Moore KL, Persaud TVN, Torchia MG. *The Developing Human: Clinically Oriented Embryology.* 10th ed. Philadelphia: Elsevier; 2015. Fig. 18.4.)

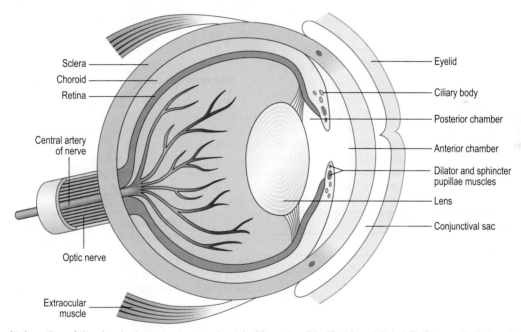

Fig. 10.14 Sagittal section of the developing eye at approximately 20 weeks. (Modified from Mitchell B, Sharma R. *Embryology: An Illustrated Colour Text.* 2nd ed. London: Elsevier; 2009.)

are formed from the posterior wall. Secondary lens fibres that are added to the external sides of the primary fibres are derived from lens equatorial cells. The primordial lens is supplied with blood by the distal part of the hyaloid artery, but the artery degenerates and the lens relies on diffusion from the aqueous and vitreous humour for nutrition.

- The pupillary membrane develops from the mesenchyme posterior to the cornea in continuity with the mesenchyme developing in the sclera.
- The primary vitreous humour is derived from mesenchyme of neural crest origin and secretes the matrix comprising the primary vitreous body. Secondary vitreous

humour is derived from the inner optic cup and surrounds the primary humour.

- The cornea is formed from surface ectoderm, mesenchyme and neural crest cells.
- The anterior chamber develops as apoptosis creates a mesenchymal space between the lens and cornea. The posterior chamber develops from a similar space between the iris and lens.
- The epithelium conjunctiva are formed from surface ectoderm, induced by the developing lens.
- The choroid and sclera are formed by mesenchyme of neural crest origin surrounding the optic cup. The earliest choroidal vascularisation begins at about week 15.

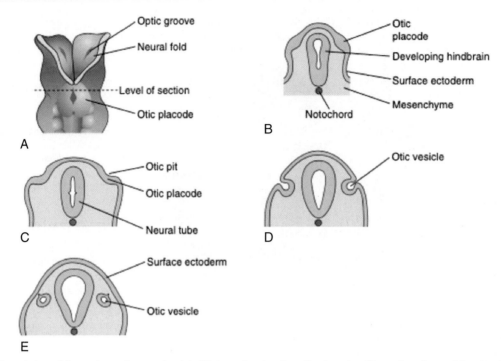

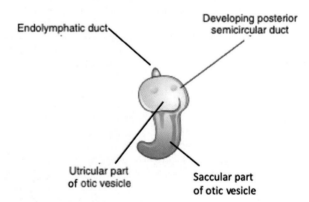

Fig. 10.15 (A) Dorsal view of the embryo at approximately 22 days showing the otic placodes. Coronal sections of the developing otic vesicle in successive stages (B), (C), (D), and (E). (Modified from Moore KL, Persaud TVN, Torchia MG. *The Developing Human: Clinically Oriented Embryology.* 10th ed. Philadelphia: Elsevier; 2015.)

- The eyelids are formed from mesenchyme (tarsal plate, levator muscle, orbicularis muscle, orbital septum and tarsal muscle) and from surface ectoderm (conjunctiva, skin epithelium, hair follicles and the glands). Fusion of the lids occurs early and but reopens by week 26 to 28.
- The lacrimal glands develop from surface ectodermal buds. At birth, the glands are small and have poor function so that neonates do not produce tears when they cry. Tears are produced in greater quantities by 1 to 3 months.

DEVELOPMENT OF THE EARS

In week 4, bilateral otic placodes develop from surface ectoderm in the region of the developing myelencephalon and invaginate, forming the otic pit and later the otic vesicle, which loses its connection to the surface ectoderm (Fig. 10.15). As a diverticulum grows from the vesicle, two regions become recognisable:

- utricular parts—dorsal region from which the endolymphatic ducts, utricles and semicircular ducts arise (Fig. 10.16);
- saccular parts—the ventral regions which produce the saccules and cochlear ducts (Fig. 10.16; see Video 10.3).

Additional diverticula bud from the utricular parts to become semicircular ducts, later enclosed in the semicircular canals of the bony labyrinth. The ampullae, within which each paired sensory cristae ampullares differentiates, develop at one end of each semicircular duct. The cochlear duct, from which the spiral organ develops, grows from the saccular part, coils and forms the membranous cochlea. The otic vesicle stimulates the surrounding mesenchyme to differentiate into a cartilaginous otic capsule which undergoes vacuolisation to form the perilymphatic space, suspending the

Fig. 10.16 Otic vesicle at approximately week 6. (Modified from Moore KL, Persaud TVN, Torchia MG. *The Developing Human: Clinically Oriented Embryology.* 10th ed. Philadelphia: Elsevier; 2015.)

labyrinth in perilymph. The perilymphatic space becomes divided into the scala tympani and scala vestibuli, whereas the otic capsule later ossifies to form the bony labyrinth.

The proximal portion of the first pharyngeal pouch forms the pharyngotympanic tube, while the distal portion expands into the tympanic cavity, housing the auditory ossicles, tendons, ligaments and the chorda tympani nerve. The malleus and incus are derived from the cartilage of the first pharyngeal arch. The crus, base of the foot plate and the head of the stapes have neural crest cell origins, whereas the outer rim of the foot plate is derived from mesodermal cells. The tensor tympani and stapedial muscles are derived from the first and second pharyngeal arches, respectively, and are innervated by the corresponding arch cranial nerve.

The external acoustic meatus also develops from the first pharyngeal groove within which ectodermal cells initially form a solid meatal plug, later degenerating to forming the internal part of the external acoustic meatus. The tympanic membrane develops from ectoderm of the first pharyngeal groove, endoderm of the tubotympanic recess and mesenchyme of the first and second pharyngeal arches. The auricle develops primarily from second arch mesenchyme with smaller contributions from the first arch.

Molecular Biology Considerations

- TGF-β family, Wnts, SHH and BMPs—differentiation of embryologic ectoderm to form the neuroplate
- SDC4 and VANGL2—neural tube closure
- SHH and Olig2 basic helix-loop-helix signalling—proliferation, survival and patterning of neuroepithelial progenitor cells
- PFN1—microfilament polymerisation within oligodendrocyte cytoskeleton
- FGF, Canonical-Wnt, retinoic acid and Fgl signalling—patterning of the midbrain and hindbrain
- Pax6—cerebellar development
- Wnt/β-catenin signalling—induction, differentiation and patterning of the hypothalamus
- Epherin-β2, FGF8, BMP4 and WNT5A—formation of the anterior lobe of the pituitary gland
- Shh signalling—cochlear induction and morphogenesis
- Forkhead transcription factors—proliferation and differentiation of retinal precursor cells
- Hh, Wnt, FGF and BMP signalling pathways—patterning of the retina
- SCF/SCFR signalling, Lhx2, Six2, Pax6 and Rax—retinal neurogenesis
- PAX6 and SOX2—induction of the lens
- PITX3, GATA3 and FOXE3—formation and differentiation of the lens fibres
- FoxL1/3, Wnt and Notch pathways, Pax2/8, Dix—development of the otic placode

CLINICAL ISSUES

SPINA BIFIDA

Spina bifida results from failure of fusion of the neural arches of the developing vertebrae and is classified according to the degree and pattern of this neural tube defect (Fig. 10.16). The associated neurological deficit is dependent on the position and extent of the defect. In spina bifida with meningocele, a meningeal cyst contains CSF and spinal cord and spinal roots are in the normal position, although there may be other spinal cord defects. In spina bifida with meningomyelocele the spinal cord or nerve roots are contained within the meningeal cyst. Most typically this lesion occurs in the lumbar or sacral regions and most are associated with an Arnold–Chiari malformation. The most severe type of spina bifida is myeloschisis in which both the neural folds and the overlying skin did not fuse, resulting in an open spinal cord represented by a flattened mass of nervous tissue. Myeloschisis usually results in permanent paralysis or weakness of the lower limbs (Fig. 10.17).

Spina bifida occulta results from minor nonfusion of the neural arch and typically occurs at L5 or S1. It is found in

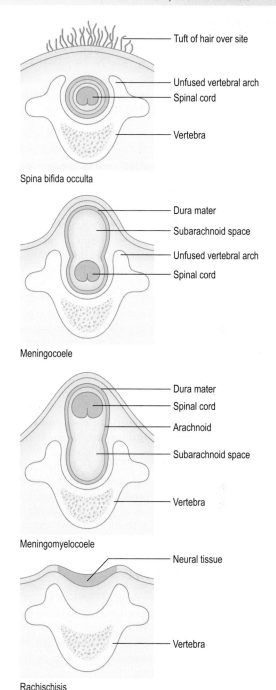

Fig. 10.17 Diagram of differing variants of spina bifida. (Modified from Mitchell B, Sharma R. *Embryology: An Illustrated Colour Text.* 2nd ed. London: Elsevier; 2009.)

approximately 10% of the population and usually produces no symptoms.

ANENCEPHALY

This severe neural tube defect results from nonclosure of the anterior neural tube. It results in absence of the calvaria, most of the brain (lacking the telencephalon), and the scalp, as well as facial defects. Most of these fetuses are stillborn whereas those born alive invariably succumb within the early neonatal period.

ENCEPHALOCELE

A defect in the formation of the cranium can result in herniation of the cranial contents, most commonly the occipital lobe of the brain. Depending on the exact location of the defect, hydrocephalus may occur, the cerebellum may herniate and a Chiari malformation may be present.

HOLOPROSENCEPHALY

Holoprosencephaly includes defects that result from failure of the cleavage of the prosencephalon. The defects may be alobar, semilobar or lobar holoprosencephaly. In the alobar form there is no falx cerebri, third ventricle, olfactory bulbs or corpus callosum, and there is a monoventricle with fused thalami. The other forms have fewer defects, but all are associated with microcephaly, anomalies of the face and varying postpartum survival.

CHIARI MALFORMATION

There are four types of Chiari malformation, all resulting from defects in the development of the cerebellum and the base of the skull (the posterior fossa is smaller than normal):

- type I—the inferior part of the cerebellum herniates through the foramen magnum, and may cause no symptoms;
- type II or Arnold–Chiari malformation—cerebellar tissue and brainstem herniate through the foramen magnum, and often accompany a myelomeningocele;
- type III—there is herniation of the cerebellum and brainstem through the foramen magnum into the vertebral canal (encephalocele containing the cerebellum);
- type IV—the cerebellum is absent or underdeveloped. These malformations may result in noncommunicating hydrocephalus.

DANDY-WALKER SYNDROME

Dandy-Walker syndrome is a group of cerebral abnormalities which include agenesis or hypoplasia of the vermis, enlargement of the posterior fossa and cystic dilation of the posterior fossa which communicating with the fourth ventricle. In almost one-half of the cases there are other neurological and nonneurological abnormalities.

SYRINGOMYELIA

Syringomyelia is a clinical disorder involving the formation of fluid-filled cysts in the spinal cord. Enlargement of the cysts may damage the spinal cord. Syringomyelia is usually associated with Chiari malformations and results from obstruction of CSF flow and accumulation (syrinx) of CSF in the spinal canal.

CRANIOPHARYNGIOMA

These are benign tumours, most commonly found in or superior to the sella turcica, that arise from epithelial remnants of the hypophyseal diverticulum. Although benign, they can be life-threatening and have a high incidence of recurrence after surgery.

ANOPHTHALMIA AND MICROPHTHALMIA

In anophthalmia, which is very rare, there is unilateral or bilateral absence of the eye and concomitant severe craniocerebral defects. This defect may be primary through failure of the optic vesicle to form, or secondary, resulting from defects in the development of the forebrain. There are many variations of microphthalmia ranging from very small eye(s) with underdeveloped face and small orbit, to situations where the eyes appear normal. The severity is related to the timing of the defect occurrence with respect to the development of various ocular structures. For instance, if the developmental error occurs before the retinal fissure closes in the sixth week, the eye may be relatively normal in size, but have gross ocular defects.

MICROTIA

Microtia results from suppressed mesenchymal proliferation within the first arch and is often a marker of other defects such as atresia of the external acoustic meatus and aural atresia. The complete absence of the auricle (anotia or grade IV microtia) is most commonly seen with first pharyngeal arch syndromes.

CONGENITAL DEAFNESS

There are many different subtypes of significant hearing loss in the neonate. Congenital impairment of hearing may be the result of maldevelopment of the components of the sound-conducting apparatus of the middle (and external ears) or of the neurosensory structures of the internal ear, as these components develop independently. Congenital deafness may be associated with first arch syndrome (malleus and incus defects) or a rubella infection resulting in defects of the spiral organ.

Case Outcome

Testing in hospital showed that EJ had elevated rubella-specific IgM titre, confirmed by reverse transcription polymer chain reaction (RT-PCR) assays and indicating a congenital rubella infection. Thirty days later, EJ met all normal mental and physical developmental milestones as assessed by his paediatrician. At 15 months of age, the parents noticed that EJ preferentially held toys to one ear. An audiology examination revealed bilateral sensory deafness.

Additional reflections: Would these results meet the criteria for congenital rubella syndrome? Why? Given the type of deafness diagnosed, what structures would have been affected by the rubella virus? How could the neonatal normal auditory brainstem response be normal, yet EJ has bilateral sensory deafness? Given this diagnosis, what might be options for EJ and his parents?

QUESTIONS

1. The epithelium of the iris develops from the:
   a. inner layer of the rim of the optic cup
   b. outer layer of the rim of the optic cup
   c. both layers of the rim of the optic cup
   d. mesenchyme near the rim of the optic cup
   e. mesenchyme between the lens and the cornea

2. Physical examination of a neonate revealed that the external acoustic meatus is atretic. This condition is the result of which of the following?
   a. Otic pit did not form
   b. Development of the first pharyngeal pouch is affected
   c. Failure of the meatal plug to canalise
   d. Auricular hillocks did not develop
   e. Tubotympanic recess has degenerated

3. Each of the following is a derivative of the alar plates except the:
   a. gracile nucleus
   b. pontine nucleus
   c. dorsal grey horn
   d. cuneate nucleus
   e. ventral grey horn

4. The pons and cerebellum are derived from the walls of the:
   a. telencephalon
   b. mesencephalon
   c. myelencephalon
   d. midbrain
   e. metencephalon

BIBLIOGRAPHY

George S, Viswanathan R, Sapkal GN. Molecular aspects of the teratogenesis of rubella virus. Biol Res 2019;52:47. doi.org/10.1186/ss40659-019-0254-3.

Manganaro L, Bernardo S, Antonelli A, et al. Fetal MRI central nervous system: State-of-the-art. Eur J Radiol 2017;93:273–83. doi: 10.1016/j.ejrad.2017.06.004.

Vasung L, Abaci Turk E, Ferradal SL, et al. Exploring early human brain development with structural and physiological neuroimaging. Neuroimage 2019;187:226–54. doi: 10.1016/j.neuroimage.2018.07.041.

11 Development of the Alimentary System

Case Scenario

PT is a 48-year-old previously healthy man who presents to the local emergency department with a 12-hour history of epigastric pain, nausea and anorexia. Abdominal examination was normal and PT was sent home with a diagnosis of gastroenteritis and recommendation for analgesia and rehydration. PT continued to have severe pain at home that evening and throughout the following day.

Questions for reflection: Considering possible congenital anomalies, what might be your differential diagnosis for PT?

DEVELOPMENT OF THE ALIMENTARY SYSTEM

During head, tail and lateral folding, the dorsal part of the umbilical vesicle becomes incorporated into the developing embryo to form the primordial alimentary tract, closed by the oropharyngeal and cloacal membranes. The endoderm of the umbilical vesicle and surrounding mesoderm form most of the gut, epithelium and glands whereas the muscular, connective tissue and other layers of the gut are derived from the surrounding splanchnic mesenchyme (see Video 11.1).

FOREGUT

The derivatives of the foregut include the pharynx, lower respiratory system, oesophagus, stomach, duodenum (proximal to the opening of the bile duct) liver, biliary apparatus and pancreas; all, except the pharynx and respiratory system, are supplied by the celiac artery. The separation of the trachea from the oesophagus by the tracheoesophageal septum is described in Chapter 9. Like many other gut derivatives, the oesophageal epithelium and glands are derived from endoderm. These epithelial cells also initially proliferate rapidly, obliterate the lumen of the oesophagus and then undergo apoptosis to create the definitive lumen. The superior part of the esophageal muscularis externa is derived from the fourth and sixth arch mesenchyme whereas the inferior part of the muscularis externa develops from the surrounding splanchnic mesenchyme.

In the fourth week, the distal foregut undergoes an initial symmetric dilation, which then becomes asymmetric owing to polarisation and radial rearrangement of the epithelium of the dorsal border of the right wall, with these cells growing faster than those on the ventral border. This asymmetric growth delineates the developing greater curvature of the stomach (Fig. 11.2A). Such differential growth results in

passive repositioning of the stomach so that the lesser and greater curvatures move to the left and right, respectively. The original left and right sides of the stomach become ventral and dorsal surfaces, respectively, and the long axis of the stomach becomes almost transverse to the long axis of the body (Fig. 11.2B). The stomach is suspended from the dorsal wall of the abdominal cavity by a dorsal mesentery, which is transposed to the left during repositioning of the stomach, forming the omental bursa. This mesentery contains the primordial spleen and the celiac artery. The suspensory ventral mesentery suspends the stomach from the ventral abdominal wall and also attaches the duodenum to the liver. Apoptotic portions of the dorsal mesenchyme form at the omental bursa (lesser peritoneal sac), which expands transversely and cranially and facilitates movements of the stomach. As the stomach enlarges, so does the dorsal mesentery to form the greater omentum, overhanging the developing intestines (Fig. 11.2B).

The duodenum forms from the caudal part of the foregut and the cranial part of the midgut, with the junction of the two parts just distal to the origin of the bile duct. The duodenum grows rapidly and as the stomach becomes repositioned, the C-shaped duodenum rotates to the right and is pressed against the posterior abdominal wall, becoming retroperitoneal. The dual derivation of the duodenum means that its vascular supply comes from branches of the both the celiac trunk and superior mesenteric arteries. The lumen of the duodenum undergoes an obliteration–recanalisation process, during which most of its ventral mesentery disappears.

The hepatic diverticulum develops from the distal portion of the foregut, between layers of the ventral mesentery (Fig. 11.3A). This diverticulum grows and divides into a larger cranial portion, the primordium of the liver, and a smaller caudal portion, the primordium of the gallbladder; the stalk of the diverticulum forms the cystic duct which joins the hepatic duct to form the bile duct. Within the developing liver, endodermal cells form anastomosing cords of hepatocytes around endothelium-lined spaces, the primordial hepatic sinusoids. Endodermal cells also give rise to the epithelial lining of the intrahepatic part of the biliary apparatus. The fibrous and haematopoietic tissue of the liver are derived from mesenchyme whereas the Kupffer cells originate from cells of the umbilical vesicle. The liver proliferates rapidly and it fills a large portion of the upper abdominal cavity; by week 9 the liver accounts for approximately 10% of the total weight of the fetus. The cholangiocytes of the extrahepatic ducts are derived from endoderm. The ventral mesentery covers the liver except for the bare area, which is in direct contact with the diaphragm.

The caudal part of the foregut also gives rise to a large dorsal and a smaller ventral pancreatic bud of endodermal cells

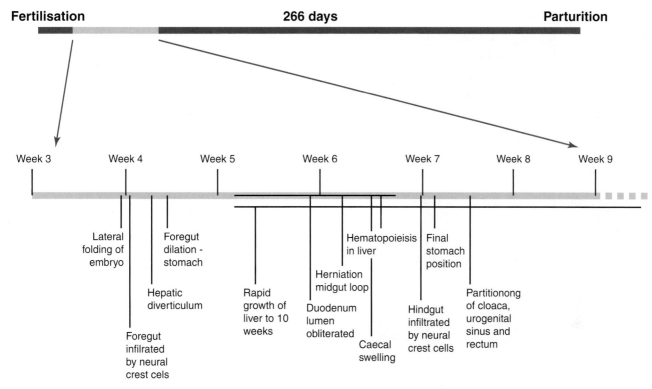

Fig. 11.1   Timeline of development related to the alimentary tract.

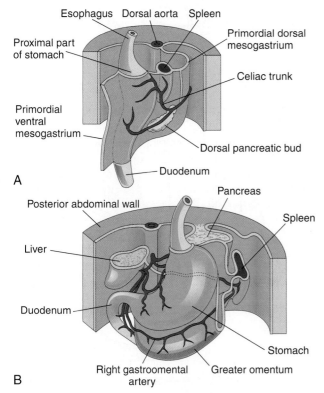

Fig. 11.2   (A) Median section of the abdomen of an embryo of approximately 35 days. (B) Embryo at 48 days. (Modified from Moore KL, Persaud TVN, Torchia MG. *The Developing Human: Clinically Oriented Embryology*. 10th ed. Philadelphia: Elsevier; 2015. Fig. 11.2.)

between the respective mesenteries (Fig. 11.3A). Repositioning of the duodenum causes the ventral pancreatic bud to be carried dorsally with the bile duct. The ventral bud comes to lie posterior to the dorsal pancreatic bud, and then fuses with it (Fig. 11.3B). The ventral pancreatic bud forms the uncinate process and part of the head of the pancreas. The pancreatic duct is created by fusion of the duct of the ventral bud and the distal part of the duct of the dorsal bud. In a minority of cases the pancreatic ducts fail to fuse, resulting in two ducts (pancreas divisum). The parenchyma of the pancreas forms from the endoderm of the buds and creates a network of tubules (primitive pancreatic ducts) around which cell clusters, primitive pancreatic acini, develop. The pancreatic islets develop from groups of cells that separate from the tubules and lie between the acini. Insulin secretion begins at approximately 10 weeks with glucagon secretion beginning a few weeks later.

During the fifth week, a mass of mesenchymal cells within the layers of the dorsal mesentery differentiate to form the capsule, connective tissue and parenchyma of the spleen. The fetal spleen is lobulated, but the lobules normally disappear before birth.

MIDGUT

The midgut includes the duodenum (distal to the opening of the bile duct), jejunum, ileum, cecum, appendix, ascending colon and right one-half to two-thirds of the transverse colon, all supplied by the superior mesenteric artery.

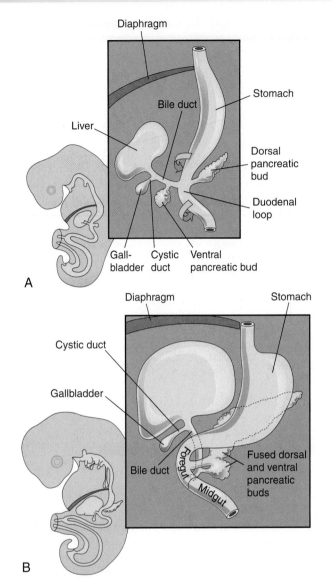

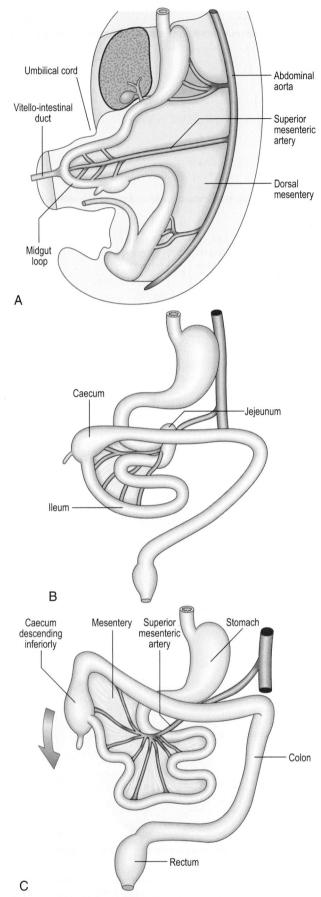

Fig. 11.3 (A) Median section of the abdomen of an embryo of approximately 35 days. (B) Embryo at 42 days. (Modified from Moore KL, Persaud TVN, Torchia MG. *The Developing Human: Clinically Oriented Embryology.* 10th ed. Philadelphia: Elsevier; 2015. Fig. 11.5.)

The midgut elongates very rapidly, forming a long loop of intestine that by week 6 herniates into the remnant of the extraembryonic coelom in the proximal part of the umbilical cord (Fig, 11.4A). The herniation occurs because of the relatively small available volume of the abdominal cavity given the large size of the liver and developing kidneys. The midgut loop has a cranial and caudal limbs which are suspended by the dorsal mesentery. The remnant of the connection of the midgut to the umbilical vesicle, the omphaloenteric duct, is attached at the apex of the midgut loop. The cranial limb of the midgut forms the small intestinal loops (ileum and jejunum) whereas the caudal limb gives rise to the caecum and appendix, the ascending colon, and a portion of the transverse colon. Differential growth during herniation of the intestines results in the cranial and caudal limbs moving to the right and left respectively (Fig. 11.4B).

The reduction of the midgut hernia begins during week 10 and is completed by the end of week 12. The small intestine returns first. The colon then reenters, pressing the duodenum and pancreas against the posterior abdominal

Fig. 11.4 (A) Median section of the abdomen of an embryo of approximately 8 weeks. (B) Embryo at 10 weeks. (C) Embryo at 14 weeks. (Adapted from Mitchell B, Sharma R. *Embryology: An Illustrated Colour Text.* 2nd ed. London: Elsevier; 2009. Figs 7.10, 7.11.)

wall causing their retroperitoneal positioning (Fig. 11.4C). As the intestines continue to lengthen, the mesentery of the ascending colon fuses with the parietal peritoneum on the dorsal abdominal wall and disappears; the ascending colon becomes retroperitoneal. Along the antimesenteric border of the midgut caudal loop, the caecal swelling appears during week 6 as the primordium of the caecum and appendix. The position of the appendix varies and may be found in retrocaecal (most common), retrocolic or pelvic positions.

HINDGUT

The left half of the transverse colon, descending and sigmoid colon, rectum and superior anal canal are all derivatives of the hindgut, as is the epithelium of the urinary bladder and most of the urethra. The part of the transverse colon derived from the midgut and that from the hindgut are demarcated by the blood supply change from a branch of the superior mesenteric artery to that of the inferior mesenteric artery, respectively. The descending colon becomes retroperitoneal when its mesentery fuses with the parietal peritoneum.

In the embryo, the hindgut and the allantois empty into the cloaca, the endodermal-lined terminus of the hindgut in contact with the surface ectoderm at the cloacal membrane (Fig. 11.5A). The cloaca becomes divided by the urorectal septum into three parts: the rectum, the cranial part of the anal canal and the urogenital sinus (Fig. 11.5B). After the cloacal membrane undergoes apoptosis the anorectal lumen is temporarily closed by an epithelial plug which degenerates to form the anal pit (proctodeum) from which the inferior anal canal develops. The hindgut origin of the superior two-thirds of the anal canal is mainly supplied by a continuation of the inferior mesenteric artery (hindgut artery) and its nerves are from the autonomic nervous

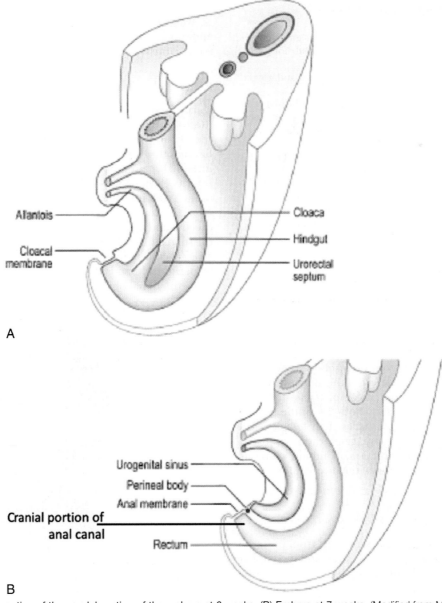

Fig. 11.5   (A) Median section of the caudal portion of the embryo at 6 weeks. (B) Embryo at 7 weeks. (Modified from Mitchell B, Sharma R. *Embryology: An Illustrated Colour Text.* 2nd ed. London: Elsevier; 2009. Fig. 7.14.)

system (ANS), whereas the inferior one-third is supplied by branches of the internal pudendal artery and its nerve supply is from the inferior rectal nerve. The junction of two sources of epithelium (ectoderm—skin; endoderm—hindgut) of the anal canal is indicated approximately by the pectinate line, located at the inferior limit of the anal valves.

ENTERIC NERVOUS SYSTEM

The enteric nervous system (ENS), comprising ganglionic plexi and enteric neurons of many subtypes, controls numerous functions of the alimentary canal including transportation, secretion, digestion and protection. The ENS is created as neural crest cells migrate to the foregut during its development. As formation of the gut continues, these neural crest cells migrate along the length of the developing gut and populate it with neurons, glial cells and other components of the ENS.

Molecular Biology Considerations

- Hox and ParaHox genes, Shh, BMP and Wnt signals—differentiation of the primordial gut into foregut, midgut, hindgut
- Foxj1, Nodal and Pitx2—left–right asymmetry and rotation of the gut
- GATA6—endoderm development and pancreas formation
- SDF1—formation and branching of the pancreatic tubules
- neurogenin 3—differentiation of pancreatic islet endocrine cells
- capsulin and homeobox genes NKx2–5, Hox11 and Bapx1—development of the spleen
- β-catenin signalling—formation of the urorectal septum.
- ISL1 (1SL LIM homeobox 1) gene—urorectal malformations
- RET and EDNRB signalling pathways—development of the enteric nervous system.

CLINICAL ISSUES

MECKEL DIVERTICULUM

Outpouching of part of the ileum (Meckel diverticulum) is the most common congenital defect of the alimentary tract. Meckel diverticulum results from incomplete closure of the omphaloenteric duct. It occurs in about 2% of the population and it is more prevalent in males than females. The Meckel diverticulum may perforate, cause diverticulitis, intestinal bleeding or bowel obstruction, or mimic symptoms of appendicitis. Surgical resection of the diverticulum is usually carried out.

OESOPHAGEAL ATRESIA

Most commonly, oesophageal atresia results from posterior deviation of the tracheoesophageal septum and incomplete separation of the oesophagus from the laryngotracheal tube. Less commonly, isolated atresia is caused by failure of recanalisation of the oesophagus.

Oesophageal atresia is associated with tracheoesophageal fistula in most cases. Polyhydramnios occurs because the fetus is unable to swallow amniotic fluid for passage to and absorption by the intestine.

HYPERTROPHIC PYLORIC STENOSIS

This is a common (1.4–4:1000; males > females) anomaly of the stomach marked by hypertrophy of the circular and longitudinal muscles of the pyloric region which results in severe stenosis of the pyloric canal. The stenosis causes obstruction of digested food, distention of the stomach with regurgitation and projectile vomiting. The cause of congenital pyloric stenosis is unknown.

ANNULAR PANCREAS

It is thought that the development of a bifid ventral pancreatic bud around the duodenum, fusing with the dorsal bud, forms a pancreatic ring. An annular pancreas may cause partial or complete duodenal obstruction that may be symptomatic in the infant or remain asymptomatic until adulthood, when duodenal obstruction can occur following pancreatitis.

INTESTINAL MALROTATION

During reduction of the physiological gut hernia and return of the intestines to the abdominal cavity, the order of reentry and position of fixation can alter the normal configuration of the intestines. In the most common form of intestinal malrotation, the caudal limb of the midgut loop returns earlier than normal, with the first returning parts of the small intestine located on the right side of the abdomen, the large intestine pushed more transversely, and the caecum and appendix located just inferior to the pylorus of the stomach (subhepatic caecum and appendix) (Fig. 11.6). The caecum is fixed to the posterolateral abdominal wall by peritoneal bands that pass over the duodenum and may cause duodenal obstruction or intestinal volvulus.

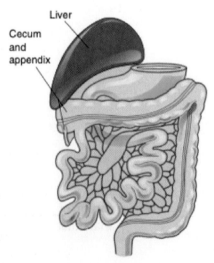

Fig. 11.6   Diagram of malrotation of the gut. (Modified from Moore KL, Persaud TVN, Torchia MG. *The Developing Human: Clinically Oriented Embryology.* 10th ed. Philadelphia: Elsevier; 2015. Fig. 11.20.)

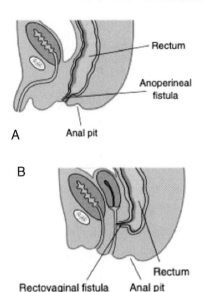

Fig. 11.7 Diagram of anorectal defects. (A) Rectal agenesis with anoperitoneal fistula. (B) Anorectal agenesis with a rectovaginal fistula. (Modified from Moore KL, Persaud TVN, Torchia MG. *The Developing Human: Clinically Oriented Embryology.* 10th ed. Philadelphia: Elsevier; 2015. Fig. 11.29.)

STENOSIS AND ATRESIA OF THE INTESTINE

Partial occlusion and atresia occur most frequently in the ileum and duodenum and result from several possible causes, including failure the gut recanalisation process in the area of obstruction or interruption of the local blood supply because of fetal distress or a volvulus. The loss of blood supply leads to necrosis of the intestine and development of a fibrous cord connecting the proximal and distal ends of the normal intestine. Gut malfixation during reduction of the midgut hernia can predispose the gut to volvulus and strangulation.

ANORECTAL ANOMALIES

Incomplete division of the cloaca by the urorectal septum is the underlying pathology in most anorectal anomalies.

Lesions are classified as low or high depending on whether the rectum ends superior or inferior to the puborectalis muscle, which maintains faecal continence and relaxes to allow defecation. In some low defects (rectum ends inferior to the puborectalis muscle) the anal canal may end blindly or there may be an ectopic anus or an anoperineal fistula that opens into the perineum—imperforate anus (Fig. 11.7A). Many low anorectal defects are associated with a fistula connecting the rectum and urethra. In other cases there is anal stenosis, which is probably caused by a dorsal deviation of the urorectal septum, or membranous atresia where the anus is in the normal position but a thin layer of tissue separates the anal canal from the exterior. High defects of the anorectal region include anorectal agenesis where the rectum ends superior to the puborectalis muscle, usually with a rectovesical, rectourethral, rectovaginal or rectovestibular fistula, depending on the sex (Fig. 11.7B). Anorectal agenesis with a fistula is caused by incomplete separation of the cloaca from the urogenital sinus. In rectal atresia, the anal canal and rectum are present but separated; the cause may be abnormal recanalisation or a defect or change of the local blood supply.

Case Outcome

Two mornings later, PT did not show up at work and a telephone call from his coworkers went unanswered over many hours. Worried that this was unusual behaviour, the coworkers contacted the brother of PT who discovered PT unconscious in his apartment. Aggressive resuscitation and treatment of septic shock was required – the patient had a ruptured subhepatic appendix and peritonitis.

Additional reflection: What alterations to the typical development of the midgut could have resulted in the appendix being located in the subhepatic region? How would the symptoms for appendicitis vary given the various possible locations for the appendix? What other disorders might appendicitis mimic?

QUESTIONS

1. Blood is supplied to the developing caudal portion of the foregut by which artery?
   a. Superior mesenteric
   b. Inferior mesenteric
   c. Dorsal aorta
   d. Intersegmental
   e. Celiac

2. The junction of the endodermal lining of the hindgut and the ectodermal epithelium of the developing anus, is approximated by the:
   a. levator ani muscle
   b. pectinate line
   c. external rectal sphincter
   d. superior limit of the anal valves
   e. urorectal septum

3. Which of the following is true regarding anorectal anomalies?

   a. The demarcation for high versus low anomalies is the pectinate line
   b. Low anomalies often include rectourethral fistula
   c. High anomalies often include an imperforate anus
   d. High anomalies include anorectal agenesis
   e. In rectal atresia, the anal canal is present, but not the rectum.

4. Which of the following statements is correct regarding development of the pancreas?
   a. The ventral pancreatic bus is formed from the foregut
   b. Insulin production begins at approximately 22 weeks
   c. The dorsal pancreatic bud is formed from the midgut
   d. The most common symptom of an annular pancreas is hyperglycaemia
   e. The dorsal pancreatic bud forms the uncinate process

BIBLIOGRAPHY

S.Y. Choi, S.S. Hong, H.J. Park, et al. The many faces of Meckel's diverticulum and its complications, J Med Imaging Radiat 61 (2017) 225–231.

N. Kruepunga, J.P.J.M. Hikspoors, H.K. Mekonen, et al. The development of the cloaca in the human embryo, J Anat 233 (2018) 724–739.

D.S. Loberbaum, L. Sussel, Gotta have GATA for human pancreas development, Cell Stem Cell 20 (2017) 577–579.

F.C. Pan, M. Brissova, Pancreas development in humans, Curr Opin Endocrinol Diabetes Obes 21 (2014) 77–82.

D.M. Popescu, R.A. Botting, E. Stephenson, et al. Decoding human fetal liver haematopoiesis, Nature 574 (2019) 365–371.

J.H.M. Soffers, J.P.J.M. Hikspoors, H.K. Mekonen, et al. The growth pattern of the human intestine and its mesentery, BMC Dev Biol 15 (2015) 31, doi: 10.1186/s12861-015-008.

P.M. Som, A. Grapin-Botton, The current embryology of the foregut and derivatives, Neurographics 6 (2016) 43–63.

M. Van Lennep, M.M.J. Singendonk, L. Dall'OGlio, et al. Oesophageal atresia, Nat Rev Dis Primers 5 (1.) (2019) doi: 10.1038/s4 1572-019-0077-0.

Development of the Urogenital System

12

Case Scenario

A neonate, delivered by caesarean section, presented with ambiguous genitalia—hypospadias and complete fusion of the labioscrotal folds.

Questions for reflection: What structure(s) do fused labioscrotal folds normally form and would this indicate an XY,46 chromosomal complement? Does the hypospadias indicate an XY,46 chromosomal complement; why? What additional testing might be required? What anomalies might be part of your differential diagnosis?

The urogenital ridge forms on each side of the dorsal aorta from the intermediate mesoderm, and can be subdivided into the nephrogenic cord (origin of the urinary system) and the gonadal ridge (origin of the genital system).

DEVELOPMENT OF THE URINARY SYSTEM

The bilateral pronephroi are rudimentary and transitory structures, which form from the nephrogenic cord at the level of the developing neck and contain a few cell clusters and tubular structures (Fig. 12.2). The associated pronephric ducts connect the pronephroi to the cloaca. Mesonephroi, also primarily transitory structures, appear at about 28 days, caudal to the pronephroi, and act as early kidneys until the metanephroi or permanent kidneys develop (see Video 12.1).

The mesonephroi contain a small number of glomeruli and tubules; the pronephric duct is utilised by the mesonephros for connection to the cloaca and becomes the mesonephric or Wolffian duct. The metanephroi develop in the fifth week from two sources: the ureteric bud –a diverticulum from the distal mesonephric duct–and the metanephrogenic blastema (a metanephric mesenchyme)

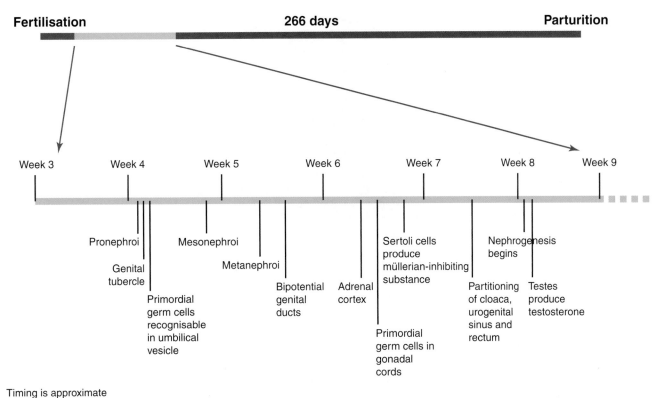

Timing is approximate

Fig. 12.1 Timeline of development related to the urogenital system.

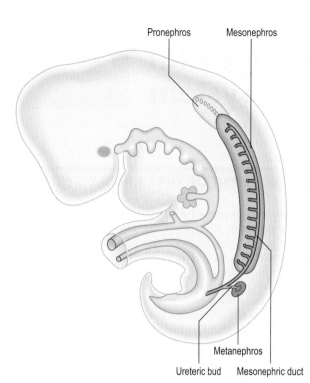

Pronephros   Mesonephros

Metanephros

Ureteric bud   Mesonephric duct

Fig. 12.2   Diagram of the three nephric structures in the fifth week. (From Mitchell B, Sharma R. *Embryology: An Illustrated Colour Text.* 2nd ed. London: Elsevier; 2009.)

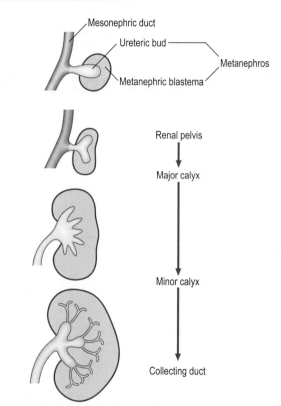

Mesonephric duct

Ureteric bud

Metanephros

Metanephric blastema

Renal pelvis

Major calyx

Minor calyx

Collecting duct

Fig. 12.3   Diagram of the branching of the ureteric bud. (From Mitchell B, Sharma R. *Embryology: An Illustrated Colour Text.* 2nd ed. London: Elsevier; 2009.)

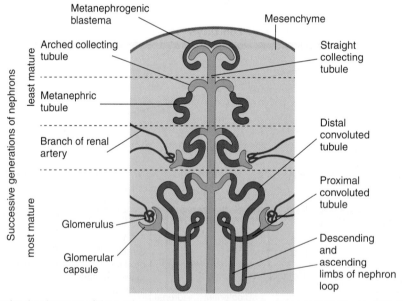

Metanephrogenic blastema

Mesenchyme

Arched collecting tubule

Straight collecting tubule

Metanephric tubule

Distal convoluted tubule

Branch of renal artery

Proximal convoluted tubule

Glomerulus

Glomerular capsule

Descending and ascending limbs of nephron loop

Successive generations of nephrons

least mature

most mature

Fig. 12.4   Diagram showing the development of the nephron. (Modified from Moore KL, Persaud TVN, Torchia MG. *The Developing Human: Clinically Oriented Embryology.* 10th ed. Philadelphia: Elsevier; 2015.)

into which the ureteric bud penetrates (Fig. 12.2). The stalk of the ureteric bud becomes the ureter. The cranial portion of the bud branches and differentiates into the collecting tubules, and minor and major calices (Fig. 12.3). The collecting tubules induce metanephrogenic blastema cells to form metanephric tubules (Fig. 12.4). Metanephric

mesenchyme condenses into cap mesenchyme from which the epithelium of the nephron is derived. The proximal ends of the metanephric tubules are invaginated by developing vascular tissue (glomeruli) while the distal portions differentiate into proximal and distal convoluted tubules; the nephron loop. The distal convoluted tubules become

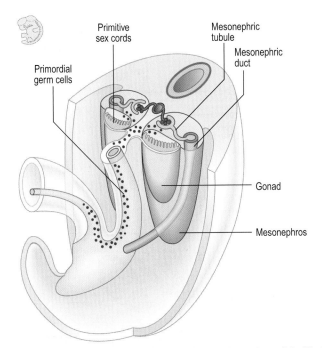

Fig. 12.5 Diagram of the transverse section of the embryo. (Modified from Mitchell B, Sharma R. *Embryology: An Illustrated Colour Text.* 2nd ed. London: Elsevier; 2009.)

confluent with a collecting tubule. Glomerular filtration begins at approximately the ninth fetal week. The number of nephrons increases rapidly reaching a maximum, 0.2 to 2.0 million in the 36th week; no new nephrons are formed beyond that time and reduced numbers may have health consequences in children and adults. Fetal kidneys are initially lobulated but this disappears in infants as the kidneys increase in size from growth of the proximal convoluted tubules and interstitial tissue.

Initially, the primordial permanent kidneys lie close to each other in the pelvis, ventral to the sacrum. Growth of the embryo and fetus results in the kidneys becoming retroperitoneal structures, located in the abdomen on either side of the vertebral column, and with the hila directed anteromedially. The source of the vascular supply of the kidneys alters as the position of the kidneys changes with embryonic development.

The epithelium of the urinary bladder develops mainly from the vesical part of the urogenital sinus (Fig. 11.5C, E) whereas other wall layers develop from splanchnic mesenchyme. Although the bladder is initially continuous with the allantois, the latter constricts and becomes the median umbilical ligament. The growth of the bladder results in the distal mesonephric ducts becoming integrated into the dorsal wall, each with a separate opening; the ducts contribute tissue to the trigone of the bladder. Repositioning of the kidneys causes the orifices of the ureters to enter obliquely through the base of the bladder. In males, the orifices enter the prostatic part of the urethra as the caudal ends of the ducts develop into the ejaculatory ducts.

The urethral epithelium is primarily derived from endoderm of the urogenital sinus, whereas the connective tissue and smooth muscle are derived from splanchnic mesenchyme. In males, the portion of the urethra in the glans penis is derived from surface ectoderm.

DEVELOPMENT OF THE GENITAL SYSTEM

Although chromosomal sex is determined at fertilisation, male and female phenotypic characteristics do not begin to appear in the embryo until the seventh week. The initial period of sex determination and development is bipotential. Development of a male phenotype requires a functional Y chromosome with the SRY gene for testis-determining factor that determines testicular differentiation. Development of the female phenotype requires two X chromosomes. A number of genes and regions of the X chromosome have special roles in sex determination. The type of gonad determines the direction of sexual differentiation that occurs in the genital ducts and external genitalia (see Video 12.2).

Proliferation of mesothelium and the underlying mesenchyme produces a bulge, the gonadal ridge, on the medial side of the mesonephros (Fig. 12.5). Gonadal epithelial cords grow into this mesenchyme resulting in the primordial bipotential gonads having an outer cortex and an inner medulla (Fig. 12.5). With an XX sex chromosome complex, the cortex of the indifferent gonad differentiates into an ovary and the medulla regresses, whereas an XY sex chromosome complex results in the medulla differentiating into a testis and the cortex regressing. Germs cells develop from endodermal cells of the umbilical vesicle and migrate along the dorsal mesentery of the hindgut to the gonadal ridges, so that by the sixth week the germ cells are incorporated in the gonadal epithelial cords (Fig. 12.5). The influence of testis-determining factor results in the gonadal cords differentiating into testicular primordial seminiferous cords tubules; without testes-determining factor, the gonad becomes an ovary under the influence of other X chromosomal factors.

With an XY chromosome complex, the primordial seminiferous cords develop into the seminiferous tubules, tubuli recti (straight tubules) and rete testis and are separated by mesenchyme that differentiates into Leydig cells. The Leydig cells begin to secrete testosterone and androstenedione during the eighth week to induce masculine differentiation of the rest of the genital system. The fetal testicular sustentacular or Sertoli cells produce müllerian-inhibiting substance (MIS) beginning in week 8, which suppresses development of the paramesonephric ducts, which would form the uterus and uterine tubes. The rete testis and mesonephric tubules become efferent ductules, connected to the mesonephric duct, which becomes the duct of the epididymis.

The gubernaculum, comprised of a linear band of mesenchymal connective tissue in the region of the mesonephros, develops with its caudal end situated at the site of the future inguinal canal. A small evagination of the lower abdominal wall, the process vaginalis, develops adjacent to the gubernaculum. The process vaginalis herniates through the wall adjacent to the caudal portion of the gubernaculum, providing a path for testicular descent into the scrotum (Fig. 12.6). The opening in the transversalis fascia, resulting from the extending process vaginalis, becomes the deep inguinal ring. The descent of the testes through the inguinal canal is a result of many factors including increasing abdominal pressure, as well as atrophy of the mesonephroi and paramesonephric ducts which allows for movement. Typically, by 26 weeks the testes have descended externally to the process

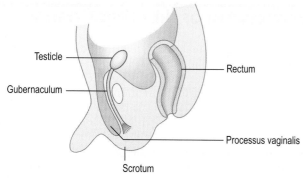

Fig. 12.6 Sagittal section of the embryo at approximately 28 weeks. (Modified from Mitchell B, Sharma R. *Embryology: An Illustrated Colour Text.* 2nd ed. London: Elsevier; 2009.)

vaginalis (retroperitoneally) to the deep inguinal ring, followed shortly by their descent into the scrotum by 32 weeks. Both testes are present in the scrotum in most fetuses. After descent, the inguinal canal contracts around the spermatic cord. Postnatally, the process vaginalis envelopes the front and sides of the testes forming the tunica vaginalis.

The ovary develops more slowly than the testes. At approximately 16 weeks, the gonadal epithelial cords break up into primordial follicles, each containing a germ cell (oogonium). The follicles are surrounded by a single layer of flattened follicular cells derived from the surface epithelium. Active mitosis of oogonia occurs during fetal life, resulting in approximately 2 million more primordial follicles, but no oogonia form postnatally. These oogonia become primary oocytes.

The inguinal canals also form in females, although as the ovaries become repositioned from the lumbar region of the posterior abdominal wall to the lateral wall of the pelvis they do not enter the inguinal canals. The gubernaculum becomes the ovarian ligament and the round ligament of the uterus, the latter passing through the inguinal canals and terminating in the labia majora. The process vaginalis is obliterated.

During the fifth week, bilateral paramesonephric (müllerian) ducts form from mesothelium of the mesonephric ducts and adjacent to the gonads and mesonephric ducts (Fig. 12.7). The cranial end of the paramesonephric ducts open into the peritoneal cavity. The mesonephric ducts play an important part in the development of the male reproductive system whereas the paramesonephric ducts are important for the development of the female reproductive system.

Testosterone induces the proximal part of the mesonephric ducts to grow, convolute and form the epididymis (Fig. 12.8). The efferent ductules open into the duct of the epididymis. Distal to the epididymis, the mesonephric duct becomes the ductus deferens. Lateral outgrowths from the caudal end of each mesonephric duct become seminal glands while the part of the duct between the entry of the seminal gland and the urethra becomes the ejaculatory duct. Multiple endodermal outgrowths arise from the prostatic part of the urethra and grow into the surrounding mesenchyme to become the prostatic glandular epithelium. The bulbourethral glands develop similarly from the spongy part of the urethra.

In embryos with XX chromosomal complement, the mesonephric ducts regress because of the absence of both testosterone and MIS. The development of the uterine tubes, uterus and superior part of the vagina is stimulated

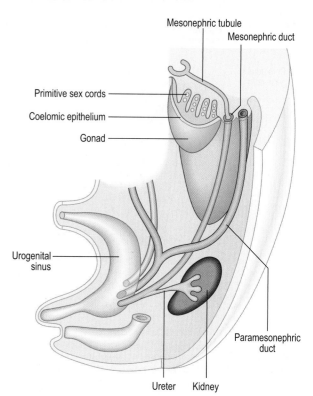

Fig. 12.7 Drawing of the ventral view of the embryo at approximately 7 weeks. (Modified from Mitchell B, Sharma R. *Embryology: An Illustrated Colour Text.* 2nd ed. London: Elsevier; 2009.)

by oestrogens from maternal ovaries and the placenta. The uterine tubes develop from the unfused cranial portions of the paramesonephric ducts while the uterus and vagina form from the caudal portions of the duct, which become fused (Fig. 12.7). Fusion of the paramesonephric ducts results in the formation of a peritoneal fold that becomes the broad ligament and the rectouterine and vesicouterine pouches. The mucus-secreting Skene's glands (urethral, paraurethral and vestibular glands) grow as outpouchings from the urethra.

The vaginal plate is derived from paired sinovaginal bulbs that grow from the location of fusion of the uterovaginal (caudal paramesonephric ducts) and the urogenital sinus (Fig. 12.8B). As the central portion of the plate undergoes apoptosis, the lumen and epithelium of the vagina are formed. The fibromuscular wall of the vagina develops from the surrounding mesenchyme.

DEVELOPMENT OF THE EXTERNAL GENITALIA

Early in week 4, proliferating mesenchyme at the cranial portion of the cloacal membrane produces the genital tubercle, which is the primordium of the penis or clitoris, depending on the sex chromosome complement. Labioscrotal swellings develop on each side of the cloacal membrane. Similar to the bipotential nature of the early gonads, the external genitalia of both sexes are similar until about the ninth week.

Under the influence of testosterone, the genital tubercle enlarges to form the penis (Fig. 12.9). On the ventral side of the developing penis, a urethral plate develops, canalises and opens to form the urethral groove, bounded by urethral folds. These urethral folds fuse in three layers: the epithelium to form the urethra; the stroma, to form part of

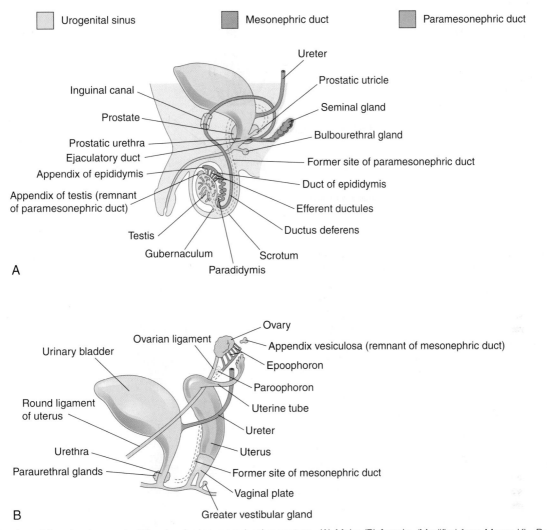

Fig. 12.8 Drawing of the development of the developing reproductive system. (A) Male; (B) female. (Modified from Moore KL, Persaud TVN, Torchia MG. *The Developing Human: Clinically Oriented Embryology.* 10th ed. Philadelphia: Elsevier; 2015.)

the penile spongiosum; and surface ectoderm to form the penile raphe and to enclose the spongy urethra within the penis. The remainder of the corpus spongiosum and the entire corpus cavernosum penis develop from mesenchyme in the phallus. Endodermal ingrowth at the tip of the glans penis meets the spongy urethra, canalises and joins the spongy urethra to form the definitive full urethra. Endoderm at the periphery of the glans penis forms the prepuce. The bilateral labioscrotal swellings fuse to form the scrotum.

In females, without the influence of testosterone, the genital tubercle becomes the clitoris. Except at the frenulum of the labia minora, the urethral folds do not fuse, but form the labia minora. The labioscrotal folds fuse anteriorly to form the mons pubis, whereas the nonfused portions form the labia majora (Fig. 12.9)

ADRENAL GLANDS

The cortex of the adrenals develops from the mesenchyme of the urogenital ridge while the medulla develops from cells of the adjacent sympathetic ganglion, originating from neural crest cells (Fig. 12.10). As the neural crest cells are enveloped by the cortex, they differentiate into the secretory cells. The zona glomerulosa and zona fasciculata are present at birth, but the zona reticularis is not recognisable until about 4 years of age. Relative to body weight, the adrenal glands of the fetus are much larger than adults because of the large fetal cortex, which produces steroid precursors for placental oestrogen. The adrenal glands rapidly regain a normal relative size during the first year of infancy.

Molecular Biology Considerations

- WT1, steroidogenic factor 1, DAX1, Sry and Sox9—genital ridge formation and differentiation
- BMP7,Wnt9b, Bmp7-SMAD and Notch/β-catenin signalling—induction of the nephron
- vHNF1 (HNF1β), Wnt1b, GDNF, Fgf10 signalling—induction and branching of the ureteric bud
- Emx2 and Pax2—control of ureteric bud branching
- Sf1, DAX1, Pbx1, GATA4 and GATA6—development of the adrenal cortex
- FOG2, WT1, NR5A1, Sry and Sox9—bipotential gonad development
- stella, fragilis, BMP4—migration of primordial germ cells.

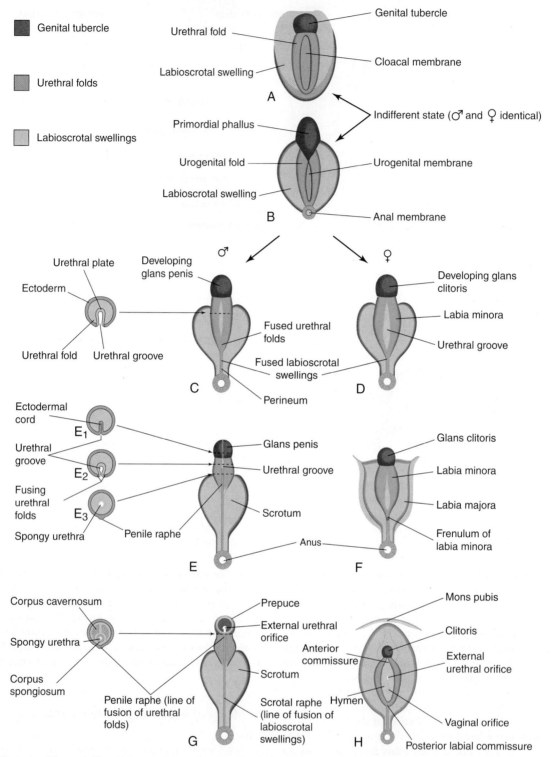

Fig. 12.9 Diagram of the early development of the external genitalia. (A, B) Appearance of genitalia during the bipotential stage (4–7 weeks). (C, E, G) Male genitalia at 9, 11, and 12 weeks. (D, F, H) Female genitalia at 9, 11, and 12 weeks. (From Moore KL, Persaud TVN, Torchia MG. *The Developing Human: Clinically Oriented Embryology.* 10th ed. Philadelphia: Elsevier; 2015.)

CLINICAL ISSUES

HYPOSPADIAS

Hypospadias, the most common defect of the penis, results from insufficient androgen production by the fetal testes. In this condition, the ectodermal portion of the urethra may fail to canalise or the fusion of the urethral folds maybe incomplete. The penis may also be underdeveloped. Together, glanular hypospadias (urethral orifice on the ventral surface of glans penis) and penile hypospadias (urethral orifice on the ventral body of the penis) make up the vast majority of cases. Less commonly, the urethral orifice is at the junction of the penis and scrotum (penoscrotal hypospadias) or between

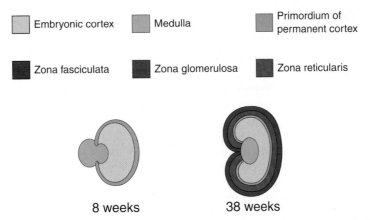

Fig. 12.10 Diagrams of the developing adrenal gland. (Modified from Moore KL, Persaud TVN, Torchia MG. *The Developing Human: Clinically Oriented Embryology.* 10th ed. Philadelphia: Elsevier; 2015.)

the unfused halves of the scrotum (perineal hypospadias), resulting from a lack of fusion of the labioscrotal folds.

EPISPADIAS

Less frequently, abnormal partitioning of the cloacal membrane with dysmorphology of the genital tubercle and its more dorsal positioning results in nonclosure of the urethral plate. As a result the urethra opens on the dorsal surface of the penis. Epispadias is often associated with exstrophy of the bladder. In males, epispadias can lead to meatal ectopy resulting in an opened, flattened mucosal strip on the dorsal surface of the penis. In females (rare), epispadias results in bifid clitoris and a cleft involving the urethra and bladder neck.

POTTER (OLIGOHYDRAMNIOS) SEQUENCE

A reduced volume of amniotic fluid may result from leakage of amniotic fluid or the lack of urine production (anuria) because of renal agenesis. Renal tubular dysgenesis, an acquired or inherited autosomal disease, impairs the development of the proximal tubules which also leads to fetal anuria. Oligohydramnios causes compression of the fetus by the uterine wall, leading to deformations such as orbital hypertelorism, low-set ears and a depressed nasal bridge. In Potter sequence, compression of the chest wall leads to pulmonary hypoplasia and early postpartum death.

HORSESHOE KIDNEY

If the lower poles of the kidneys fuse in early development, a single large U-shaped kidney is found below the level of the inferior mesenteric artery or in the pelvis. A horseshoe kidney is of little physiological consequence and may go undetected because it has normal nephron function and a normal collecting system and the ureters enter the bladder.

UNILATERAL RENAL AGENESIS

In such cases, the left kidney is usually absent owing to errors in the interaction between the ureteric bud and the metanephrogenic blastema. Unilateral renal agenesis often causes no symptoms early as the other kidney can undergoes

hypertrophy and compensate for the function of the missing kidney. Long-term consequences may include hypertension.

MULTICYSTIC DYSPLASTIC KIDNEY DISEASE

Multicystic dysplastic kidney (MCDK) disease is one of the most commonly occurring diseases in children. In MCKD multiple noncommunicating cysts are present in the normal parenchyma of the kidney. The kidney collecting tubules undergo cystic dilation and little or no parenchyma may form. This disease usually affects one kidney (unilateral), causing atresia of the proximal ureter and renal pelvis.

DUPLEX COLLECTING SYSTEM

Abnormal division of the ureteric bud results in a divided kidney with a bifid ureter or a double kidney with a bifid or separate ureters.

POSTERIOR URETHRA VALVES

A complete or partial obstruction of the posterior urethra is present because of development of excess tissue, commonly where the mesonephric ducts joins the cloacal membrane. This blockage causes hydronephrosis, a trabeculated bladder, oligohydramnios, dilated ureters and renal dysplasia.

UNDESCENDED AND ECTOPIC TESTES

Cryptorchidism (undescended testes), which may be unilateral or bilateral, occurs in about 3% to 5% of full-term males. Although the testes may be in the abdominal cavity or anywhere along the usual path of descent of the testis, they are usually located in the inguinal canal. Typically, the testes descend into the scrotum by 12 months of age. If bilateral cryptorchidism is uncorrected, infertility is common. There is also a significantly higher risk of germ cell testicular tumours in abdominal cryptorchidism, so orchiopexy is required.

Rarely, the testes deviate from the normal path to locate in other ectopic locations: interstitial (external to the aponeurosis of the external oblique muscle; most common), proximal medial thigh, to the opposite side or dorsal to the penis.

DISORDERS (DIFFERENCES) OF SEXUAL DIFFERENTIATION

In these complex disorders there is a discrepancy between the morphology of the gonads and the appearance of the external genitalia. A disorder of sexual differentiation (DSD) can be classified as:

- Sex chromosome DSD—embryos with abnormal sex chromosome complexes, such as XXX, XXY or XO. If a normal Y chromosome is present, the embryo develops as a male. If no Y chromosome is present or the testis-determining region of the Y chromosome is absent, female development occurs. Two X chromosomes are needed, however, to bring about normal ovarian development although germ cells have been found in XO gonads.
- Gonadal dysgenesis—caused by inadequate production of testicular testosterone and MIS:
  - Ovotesticular DSD—both testicular and ovarian tissue in one (ovotestis) or opposite typically nonfunctioning gonads. A majority of persons with ovotesticular DSD are 46,XX with the remainder being 46,XX/46,XY mosaics or 46,XY. The causes of ovotesticular DSD are still poorly understood. The gonads are almost always nonfunctional. Although the phenotype may be male or female, the external genitalia are ambiguous.
  - XX testicular DSD—individuals with this DSD are 46,XX but have the SRY gene translocated on one X chromosome. These individuals typically have a male appearing external genitalia with small testes. Hypospadias or ambiguous genitalia may also be present.
  - XY gonadal dysgenesis—individuals with this DSD have a 46,XY chromosome constitution with variably developed external and internal genitalia because of differing degrees of development of the paramesonephric ducts.
- Virilising congenital adrenal hyperplasia (CAH) —a result of autosomal defects in the synthesis of adrenal steroids; in most cases because of a deficiency of 21-hydroxylase. This enzyme deficiency causes reduced mineralocorticoid and glucocorticoid production resulting in the pituitary gland increasing production of ACTH. Increased ACTH leads to overproduction of androgens by the adrenal gland. In females this can cause masculinisation of the external genitalia, including clitoral hypertrophy, partial fusion of the labia majora and a persistent urogenital sinus. Later in childhood, excess androgen leads to rapid growth and accelerated skeletal maturation. Males with CAH have normal external genitalia so that CAH may go undetected until rapid maturation begins. In either sex, there may also be insufficient production of aldosterone leading to salt wasting, which may present as shock from dehydration.
- Disorders of androgen action—Individuals with complete androgen insensitivity syndrome are 46,XY and have testicles, but appear as normal females. The external genitalia are female, the vagina often ends in a blind pouch and the uterus and uterine tubes are absent or rudimentary. At puberty, there is normal development of breasts and female characteristics, but without menstruation. The testes are usually in the abdomen or inguinal canals or within the labia majora. This syndrome results from a resistance to the effects of testosterone at the cellular level in the genital tubercle and labioscrotal and urethral folds. Individuals with partial androgen insensitivity syndrome exhibit some masculinisation at birth and may have an enlarged clitoris. In either situation, the testes are usually resected because approximately 30% will develop malignancy by age 50 years.

MAYER–ROKITANSKY–KÜSTER–HAUSER SYNDROME

Incomplete development of the caudal portions of the paramesonephric duct in females with 46,XX complement and normal ovaries results in underdevelopment or absence of the uterus and the upper portion of the vagina.

SEPTATE AND BICORNATE UTERI, AND UTERUS DIDELPHYS

Various types of uterine configurations can occur as a results of anomalous paramesonephric duct development or fusion:

- uterus didelphys (double uterus)—failure of fusion of the most inferior parts of the paramesonephric ducts
- septate uterus—partial fusion of the paramesonephric ducts
- bicornate uterus—lack of fusion of the more proximal portion of the paramesonephric ducts
- unicornuate uterus—one paramesonephric duct fails to develop.

Case Outcome

The neonate was in no distress and further physical examination by the paediatrician revealed no other concerns beyond those of the genitourinary system. The labioscrotal folds showed rugae and there was a urethral opening approximately 3 mm from the clitorophalus. No gonads could be palpated. A pelvic ultrasound scan identified a uterus. An ACTH (cosyntropin) stimulation test was abnormal.

Additional reflections: What is the likely diagnosis for this infant? What, if any, additional testing might be required? What treatments, if any, may be required? What might be some of the longer-term medical and quality of life concerns? What other expertise should be sought in the care of this infant and support of the parents?

QUESTIONS

1. Primordial germ cells are first seen in the fourth week within which of these structures?
   a. Wall of the allantois
   b. Gonadal ridges
   c. Umbilical vesicle
   d. Primary sex cords
   e. Dorsal mesentery

2. The ureteric bud is derived from the:
   a. urogenital sinus
   b. somatic mesoderm
   c. splanchnic mesoderm
   d. paramesonephric duct
   e. mesonephric duct

3. A bicornate uterus results from:
   a. failure of fusion of the paramesonephric ducts
   b. absence of the urogenital sinus
   c. failure of fusion of the sinovaginal bulbs
   d. incomplete formation of the urorectal septum
   e. failure of fusion of mesonephric ducts

4. Which of the following is a result of inadequate production of testicular testosterone and müllerian-inhibiting substance?
   a. Sex chromosome disorder of sexual differentiation (DSD)
   b. Congenital adrenal hyperplasia
   c. Potter sequence
   d. Androgen insensitivity syndrome
   e. Ovotesticular DSD

BIBLIOGRAPHY

A. Bashamboo, C. Eozenou, S. Rojo, et al. Anomalies in human sex determination provide unique insights into the complex genetic interactions of early gonad development, Clin Genet 91 (2017) 143–156.

A. Bashamboo, K. McElreavey, Mechanisms of sex determination in humans: insights from disorders of sex development, Sex Dev 10 (2016) 313–325.

A.P. McMahon, Development of the mammalian kidney, Curr Top Dev Biol 117 (2016) 31–64.

L.L. O'Brien, Nephron progenitor cell commitment: striking the right balance, Semin Cell Dev Biol 91 (2019) 94–103.

L.L. O'Brien, A.P. McMahon, Induction and patterning of the metanephric nephron, Semin Cell Dev Biol 36 (2014) 31–38.

S. Sharma, J. Wistuba, T. Pock, et al. Spermatogonial stem cells: updates from specification to clinical relevance, Human Reprod Update 25 (2019) 275–297.

Z.Y. She, W.X. Yang, Sry and Sox E genes: How they participate in mammalian sex determination and gonadal development?, Semin Cell Dev Biol 63 (2017) 13–22.

13 Development of Skeletal, Muscular and Integumentary Systems

Case Scenario

LE is a 36-year-old mother of two healthy children and she is now 18 weeks pregnant. Polyhydramnios was present on antenatal ultrasound, and the fetal head circumference was larger than expected, whereas fetal femur length was reduced for the given gestational age.

Questions for reflection: What might cause the reduced femur length? Could this be a result of placental insufficiency or intrauterine growth restriction? What neurological conditions might result from an enlarged head? Why would the growth curve trajectory for the head and the femur be discordant?

SKELETAL SYSTEM

At the end of the third week, the paraxial mesoderm condenses and subdivides into somites, cuboidal segmental elevations along the dorsolateral surface of the embryo (Figs. 13.1 and 13.2A). Cells within the somites are organised into two regions: the sclerotome, which forms the mesenchymal tissue that forms cartilage and bones of the axial skeleton, and the dorsolaterally located dermomyotome, which forms muscle cells and the dermis (Fig. 13.2B). The mesenchyme that gives rise to the appendicular skeleton originates from the lateral mesoderm.

DEVELOPMENT OF CARTILAGE AND BONE

During the fifth week, mesenchymal tissue condenses, and the cells differentiate into prechondrocytes and then into chondroblasts. The chondroblasts secrete the components of the extracellular matrix including proteoglycans, collagen and elastin, combinations of which create hyaline cartilage, fibrocartilage and elastic cartilage. Bone typically develops within either mesenchyme or cartilage but can also develop in tendons (sesamoid bones).

Intramembranous ossification occurs directly in mesenchyme that has become condensed and vascularised.

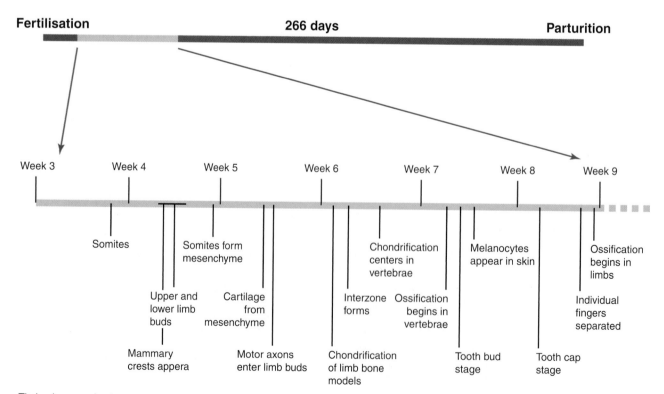

Timing is approximate

Fig. 13.1 Timeline of development related to the skeletal, muscular and integumentary systems.

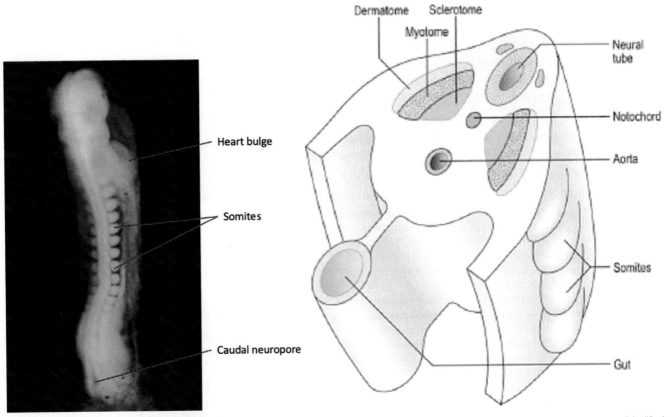

Fig. 13.2 (A) Dorsal view of an embryo at approximately 24 days showing 13 pairs of somites. (B) Transverse section of the embryo. (Modified from Moore KL, Persaud TVN, Torchia MG. *The Developing Human: Clinically Oriented Embryology*. 10th ed. Philadelphia: Elsevier; 2015 and Mitchell B, Sharma R. *Embryology: An Illustrated Colour Text*. 2nd ed. London: Elsevier; 2009.)

Mesenchymal cells differentiate into osteoblasts and deposit osteoid the unmineralised combination of type I collagen and mucopolysaccharide. Calcium phosphate is then deposited in the osteoid, trapping osteoblasts which then differentiate into osteocytes. Slowly, microscopic spicules of bone coalesce into lamellae; concentric lamellae form around blood vessels creating osteons. Peripheral osteoblasts continue to build lamellae, forming plates of compact bone on the surfaces. Between the plates, the intervening bone remains spiculated within which the mesenchyme differentiates into bone marrow.

Endochondral ossification occurs within predeveloped cartilaginous models. For instance, in a long bone, the primary centre of ossification appears in the diaphysis. Here, the chondrocytes hypertrophy, create extracellular matrix which becomes calcified and undergo apoptosis (Fig. 13.3A). The hypertrophic chondrocytes express a chemotactic factor, vascular endothelial growth factor, which attracts haematopoietic progenitor cells and endothelial cells. A thin layer of bone is deposited under the primordial periosteum (perichondrium) surrounding the diaphysis. Invasion by vascular connective tissue from blood vessels surrounding the periosteum begins to break up the cartilage model. Osteoblasts reach the developing bone from these blood vessels. Secondary ossification centres in the epiphyses arise mostly during the first few years of infancy. The epiphyseal cartilage cells undergo the same hypertrophic process but ossification spreads radially rather than longitudinally in the diaphysis (Fig. 13.3B). Lengthening of long bones occurs at the diaphyseal–epiphyseal junction where chondrocytes proliferate. Over time, the articular cartilage remains intact while the epiphyseal cartilage plate becomes replaced by spongy bone and halts any further elongation of the bone (usually by age 20 years). The development of irregular bones through endochondral ossification is similar to that in long bones except ossification begins centrally and spreads in all directions.

DEVELOPMENT OF JOINTS

Within the cartilage model, cells begin to flatten and form a separation at the location of the joint, the interzone tissue. Depending on the joint type, the interzonal cells differentiate into dense fibrous tissue, hyaline cartilage or fibrocartilage. At sites of synovial joint development, the peripheral interzone forms the joint capsule and ligaments. The central interzone undergoes cavitation to become the synovial cavity and also to produce the synovial membrane that lines the joint and articular surfaces.

DEVELOPMENT OF THE AXIAL SKELETON

With differential growth of the embryo, each somite contributes sclerotome cells that surround the notochord and neural tube. Within each segment there are more loosely arranged cells cranially and densely packed cells caudally (Fig. 13.4). Some densely packed cells fuse with the loosely arranged cells of the immediately caudal sclerotome to form the primordium of the vertebral body. The notochord degenerates where it is surrounded by the developing vertebral bodies, but between the vertebrae the notochord expands to form the nucleus pulposus of the intervertebral disc. The nucleus pulposus is later surrounded by fibres originating from the densely packed cells of the sclerotome to form the annulus fibrosus; together, the nucleus and annulus fibrosus form the intervertebral discs. The mesenchymal cells that surround the neural tube form the neural or vertebral arch. Adjacent mesenchymal cells in the body wall form the ribs in the thoracic region.

Chondrification of each mesenchymal vertebra occurs in two centres which fuse, at the end of the embryonic period, to form a cartilaginous centrum. The centres in the neural arches fuse together and with the centrum. The spinous and transverse processes develop from extension of chondrification centres in the neural arch.

The centrum ossifies through three primary centres: one in the centrum and one in each half of the neural arch. The bony halves of the vertebral arch usually fuse during the first 3 to 5 years and their articulation with the centrum allows for spinal cord growth. Secondary ossification centres appear in the vertebrae after puberty.

Ribs develop from the mesenchymal costal processes of the thoracic vertebrae. The sternum develops from individual cartilaginous sternal bars that develop ventrolaterally in the body wall, and fuse to form the manubrium, sternebrae and xiphoid process. Ossification occurs in the sternum in utero. The xyphoid does not ossify until adulthood and may remain partially cartilaginous.

The cranium consists of the neurocranium, enclosing the brain, and the viscerocranium, the facial skeleton that is derived from the pharyngeal arches. The bones in the base of the neurocranium form by fusion of several cartilages, which later undergo endochondral ossification:

- Occipital bone—the cartilage surrounding the cranial end of the notochord combines with that from the sclerotome regions of the occipital somites
- Sphenoid—the cartilage around the developing pituitary gland combined with that from the ala orbitalis
- Ethmoid—cartilage of the trabeculae cranii anterior to the developing pituitary, and from the nasal sacs

The other bones of the calvaria form by intramembranous ossification and are initially separated by six fibrous joints or sutures; fontanelles are areas where multiple sutures meet. The softness of the bones and their loose connections at the sutures enable the fetal calvaria to undergo moulding during birth.

The mesenchyme that supplies cells for the formation of the viscerocranium is derived from neural crest cells that migrate into the pharyngeal arches (See Chapter 9). The following bones are formed by endochondral ossification of pharyngeal arch cartilage: malleus, incus, portion of the stapes, styloid process of the temporal bone and the hyoid. Intramembranous ossification forms the squamous temporal, maxillary, zygomatic bones and mandible. Some endochondral ossification occurs in the median plane of the chin and the mandibular condyle.

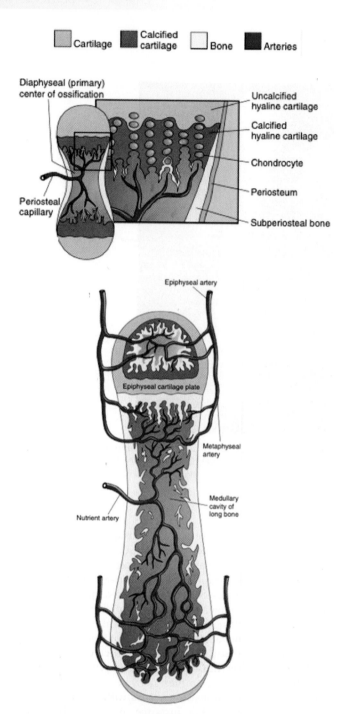

Fig. 13.3 (A) and (B) Schematic drawings of endochondral bone formation. (Modified from Moore KL, Persaud TVN, Torchia MG. *The Developing Human: Clinically Oriented Embryology*. 10th ed. Philadelphia: Elsevier; 2015.)

DEVELOPMENT OF THE APPENDICULAR SKELETON

The clavicle develops by intramembranous ossification, although it forms cartilage models at the diapheses. The cartilage models of the pectoral girdle and upper limb bones appear slightly before those of the pelvic girdle and lower limb bones. Primary ossification begins in almost all of the long bones by the end of week 11, whereas most secondary ossification centres do not appear until after birth.

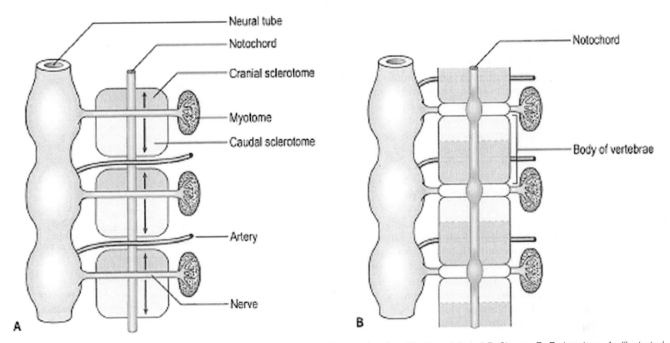

Fig. 13.4 Diagrammatic frontal sections of the embryo. (A) 4 weeks; (B) 5 weeks. (Modified from Mitchell B, Sharma R. *Embryology: An Illustrated Colour Text.* 2nd ed. London: Elsevier; 2009.)

LIMB DEVELOPMENT

Bilateral limb buds develop opposite the caudal cervical segments (upper limb buds) and opposite the lumbar and upper sacral segments (lower limb buds). The upper and lower limb buds can be seen by days 24 and 26, respectively. The ectoderm at the apex of each limb bud forms an apical ectodermal ridge (AER), composed of specialised multilayered epithelial cells. The AER initiates growth and development of the limbs, through mesenchyme proliferation in a proximodistal axis. Mesenchymal cells aggregate at the posterior margin of the limb bud to form the zone of polarising activity (ZPA) which helps to control anterior–posterior axis orientation. The mesenchyme adjacent to the AER consists of a pool of undifferentiated, rapidly proliferating cells, whereas those proximal to the AER differentiate into blood vessels and cartilage bone models. Over time the distal ends of the limb buds flatten into hand plates and foot plates which condense to outline the pattern of the digits and are separated by intervening loose mesenchyme (Fig. 13.4). These intervening regions undergo apoptosis to form notches and then separate digits. The AER at the tip of each digital ray induces development of the mesenchyme of the phalanges (See Video 13.1).

Chondrification of limb bone mesenchyme appears during week 5, and by the end of the sixth week, the entire limb skeleton is cartilaginous. Primary ossification centres are present in all long bones by the 12th week. The mesenchyme in the limb bud also gives rise to ligaments and blood vessels.

Myogenic precursor cells from the somite dermomyotomes migrate into the limb buds and differentiate into myoblasts. The myoblast aggregate adjacent to the developing bones to form muscle masses with separate extensor and flexor components. The synovial joints can be identified during week 9 (Fig. 13.5).

Innervation of the limbs begins when motor axons from the spinal cord enter the limb buds and grow into the dorsal and ventral muscle masses. Sensory axons follow the path of the motor axons. The spinal nerves are distributed in segmental bands from the somites, and supply the dorsal and ventral surfaces of the limbs, forming the dermatomes. The original dermatomal pattern evolves and overlaps somewhat attributed to growth of the limbs.

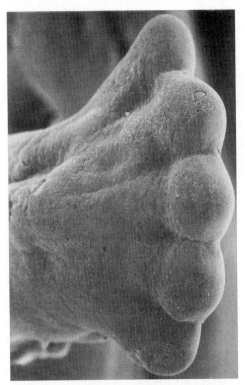

Fig. 13.5 Scanning electron micrograph of embryo foot at approximately 8 weeks. (Modified from Moore KL, Persaud TVN, Torchia MG. *The Developing Human: Clinically Oriented Embryology.* 10th ed. Philadelphia: Elsevier; 2015.)

The limb buds are initially supplied with blood by branches of the intersegmental arteries from the dorsal aorta. The earliest vascular pattern consists of a primary axial artery and branches draining into a peripheral marginal sinus, which enters a peripheral vein. The process of angiogenesis provides the source and patterning of the evolving limb vasculature. The upper limb primary axial artery becomes the brachial artery and the common interosseous artery, whereas the lower limb primary artery becomes the profunda femoris artery and the anterior and posterior tibial arteries.

DEVELOPMENT OF THE MUSCULAR SYSTEM

SKELETAL MUSCLE

Muscle development begins with the formation of myoblasts from mesenchyme; the nuclei and cell bodies elongate and then fuse to form multinucleated myotubes. Myofilaments and myofibrils develop in the cytoplasm of the myotubes, which are segregated from the surrounding connective tissue by external laminae. Fibroblasts produce the perimysium and epimysium layers of the fibrous sheath of the muscle; the endomysium is formed by the external lamina and reticular fibres. Fetal muscle growth is attributed to the ongoing fusion of myoblasts and myotubes. Most skeletal muscles develop before birth with the remainder forming before 1 year of age. Muscle growth after that time results from increased fibre diameter from formation of more myofilaments.

Each somite myotome divides into epaxial (dorsal) and hypaxial (ventral) divisions which are supplied by the spinal nerve from the dorsal and ventral primary rami, respectively (see Fig. 13.6). Epaxial division myoblasts from cervical somites form extensor muscles of the neck and vertebral column, while hypaxial divisions of the cervical myotomes form the scalene, prevertebral, geniohyoid and infrahyoid muscles. Other regional myotomes form flexor muscles of the vertebral column (thoracic myotomes), quadratus lumborum (lumbar myotomes), muscles of the pelvic diaphragm, and striated muscles of the anus and sex organs (sacrococcygeal myotomes).

SMOOTH MUSCLE

For the most part, smooth muscle arises from splanchnic and somatic mesenchyme, although muscles of the iris, and glandular myoepithelial cells, are thought to be derived from mesenchymal cells that originate from ectoderm (neural crest origin). Smooth muscle development begins with the differentiation of myoblasts from mesenchyme and development of elongated nuclei in spindle-shaped myoblasts. Unlike skeletal muscle, the myoblasts do not fuse. As smooth muscle cells (fibres) differentiate, nonsarcomeric contractile elements develop in their cytoplasm and the external surface of each cell acquires a surrounding external lamina. The fibres develop into sheets or bundles and receive autonomic innervation. Muscle cells and fibroblasts synthesise collagenous, elastic and reticular fibres. Later expansion of myoblast population occurs through division of the existing myoblasts.

DEVELOPMENT OF CARDIAC MUSCLE

Cardiac myoblasts develop from mesenchyme surrounding the early heart; this mesenchyme originates in the lateral splanchnic mesoderm. Immunohistochemical studies have

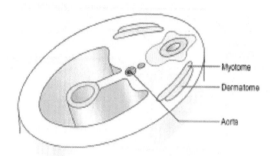

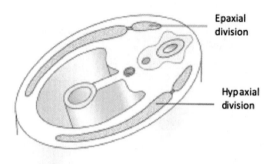

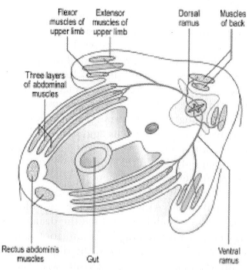

Fig. 13.6 Transverse section of the embryo showing skeletal muscle development. (Modified from Mitchell B, Sharma R. *Embryology: An Illustrated Colour Text.* 2nd ed. London: Elsevier; 2009.)

revealed a spatial distribution of tissue-specific antigens (myosin heavy-chain isoforms) in the embryonic cardiac cells between the fourth and eighth weeks. Cardiac muscle fibres arise by differentiation and growth of single cells that adhere to each other, although the intervening cell membranes do not disintegrate as in skeletal muscle. These areas of adhesion produce the intercalated discs. Growth of cardiac muscle results from the formation of new myofilaments. A special population of cardiac muscle cells (Purkinje fibres) develop from trabeculated myocardium that has fast-conducting gap junctions with relatively few myofibrils and relatively larger diameters.

DEVELOPMENT OF THE INTEGUMENTARY SYSTEM

SKIN

The skin develops from both ectoderm (epidermis) and mesenchyme (dermis). In the early embryo, the epidermis is a single layer of cuboidal ectodermal cells. By the end of week 6, the cells differentiate to form the periderm (outer layer of simple squamous epithelium) and a basal layer or basement membrane zone (collagen fibres and laminin). Peridermal cells undergo keratinisation, followed by desquamation, to then be replaced by cells from the basal layer. The desquamated peridermal cells contribute to the vernix caseosa that protects the fetal skin from exposure to amniotic fluid. Further development and differentiation of cells in the basal layer results in formation of the stratum germinativum which then produces the intermediate layer contributing to the formation of the mature keratinised epidermis. By approximately week 21, the periderm is replaced by the stratum corneum (Fig. 13.7). The stratum germinativum cells also extend into the dermis, forming epidermal ridges; by week 20, these ridges have been permanently established and have formed the fingerprint and footprint patterns. Neural crest derived melanoblasts migrate into the developing dermis, then to the dermatoepidermal junction, where they form melanocyte-associated pigment granules. The melanocytes begin producing melanin before birth and distribute it to the epidermal cells.

The dermis develops from mesenchyme, originating from somatic mesoderm and somite dermatomes. By 11 weeks, the mesenchymal cells produce collagenous and elastic connective tissue fibres. The dermis also forms dermal papillae, which interdigitate with the epidermal ridges and house either capillary loops or sensory nerve endings (Fig. 13.7). Further expansion of the dermal vasculature occurs through angiogenesis; in some capillaries mesenchymal differentiation provides muscular coats with the vessels becoming arterioles, arteries, venules and veins.

Sebaceous glands begin as cellular buds that develop from the epidermal root sheaths of hair follicles (Fig. 13.8). The buds form alveoli and ducts as they invade the dermis. Sebaceous glands independent of hair follicles, such as those of the glans penis and labia minora, develop as cellular buds from the epidermis that invade the dermis. Eccrine sweat glands develop as buds from the epidermis that grow into the underlying mesenchyme (Fig. 13.8). The extended buds form coiled ends, the bodies of the secretory parts of the glands.

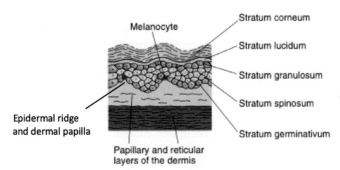

Fig. 13.7 Diagram of the layers of the skin. (Modified from Moore KL, Persaud TVN, Torchia MG. *The Developing Human: Clinically Oriented Embryology*. 10th ed. Philadelphia: Elsevier; 2015.)

The peripheral cells of the secretory parts of the glands differentiate into myoepithelial and secretory cells. The original epidermal attachment undergoes canalisation to form sweat ducts. Apocrine sweat glands form from down growths of the stratum germinativum, and therefore do not open on the skin surface, but rather into the canals of the hair follicles. Unlike eccrine sweat glands, secretion by apocrine sweat glands is influenced by hormones and does not begin until puberty.

MAMMARY GLANDS

Mammary gland development is similar in male and female embryos. Mammary crests develop from mesenchyme along each side of the ventral surface of the embryo and extend from the axillary to the inguinal region. Most of the mammary crest undergoes degeneration except at the site of the future breasts. In the remaining crests, primary mammary buds grow from epidermis into the mesenchyme, divide into several secondary mammary buds and develop into lactiferous ducts and branches. Bud canalisation is induced by placental sex hormones entering the fetal circulation. The budding-canalisation process produces approximately 15 to 19 lactiferous ducts. Breast connective tissue, fat and smooth muscle fibres of the nipple and areola are derived from mesenchyme.

Late in the fetal period, the epidermis at the site of origin of the mammary glands forms shallow mammary pits. Only after birth do the nipples elevate from the mammary pits as a result of proliferation of areolar connective tissue. Early mammary glands of male and female neonates are identical. Circulating maternal hormones may cause transitory mammary gland enlargement and galactorrhoea. In females, the breasts enlarge rapidly during puberty mainly because of development of the mammary gland tissue and the accumulation of the fibrous stroma and fat.

HAIR

Hair buds form as outgrowths of the stratum germinativum and differentiate into hair bulbs, the early hair root (Fig. 13.8). The hair bulbs provide epithelial cells for the germinal matrix, the structure that forms the shaft of the hair. The peripheral cells of these developing hair follicles form epithelial root sheaths, and the surrounding mesenchymal cells differentiate into the dermal root sheaths. Melanoblasts migrate into the hair bulbs, differentiate into melanocytes, and transfer melanin into the germinal matrix cells. The germinal matrix cells proliferate and are pushed towards the surface, where they become keratinised to form hair shafts. Arrector muscles differentiate from the mesenchyme surrounding the hair follicles and attach to the dermal root sheaths and the papillary layer of the dermis. Hair development begins early in the fetal period and hairs are first recognisable on the eyebrows, upper lip and chin. Early hair is fine and lightly pigmented but is replaced by coarser hairs during the perinatal period.

NAILS

Nail fields develop as epidermis thickenings at the tip of each digit and migrate onto the dorsal surfaces of the digit, bringing nerves from the ventral surface. Nail folds surround and then cover the nail field, later becoming keratinised to

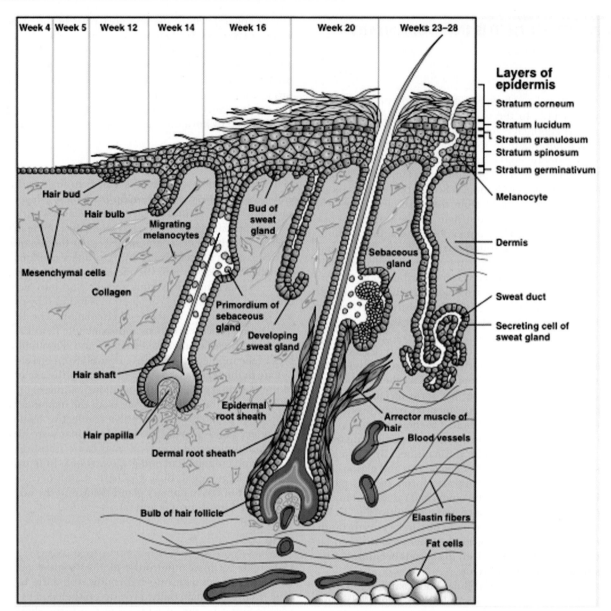

Fig. 13.8   Development of skin glands and hairs. (Modified from Moore KL, Persaud TVN, Torchia MG. *The Developing Human: Clinically Oriented Embryology*. 10th ed. Philadelphia: Elsevier; 2015.)

form the nail plate. The early nail is covered by the eponychium, which later degenerates, remaining only as the cuticle.

TEETH

During week 6, dental laminae form as U-shaped thickenings of the oral epithelium, aligned with the curvatures of the embryonic jaws. Formation of the teeth is described in four stages:

- Bud stage—In both the mandibular and maxilary dental laminae 10 tooth buds develop which grow into the underlying mesenchyme to form the deciduous teeth. Additional buds for the permanent teeth appear later in the fetal period and lingual to the deciduous tooth buds. Buds for the second and third permanent molars develop after birth.
- Cap stage—The tooth buds are invaginated by mesenchyme. The internal part of each dental papilla (cap-shaped tooth) becomes the dentin and dental pulp (Fig. 13.9). The enamel organ is formed from ectodermal cells from the dental lamina and is comprised of three layers: the outer

and inner enamel epithelium and the loosely arranged enamel reticulum in between (Fig. 13.9). Mesenchyme surrounding the developing tooth forms the vascularised dental follicle, which will differentiate into the cement. The periodontal ligament is derived from neural crest cells.
- Bell stage—The mesenchymal cells in the dental papilla, adjacent to the internal enamel epithelium, differentiate into odontoblasts, produce predentin and deposit it adjacent to the epithelium. The predentin calcifies and becomes dentin. The odontoblasts regress as the dentin thickens, although their cytoplasmic odontoblastic processes remain embedded. The increase in dentin reduces the pulp cavity to a narrow root canal through which the vessels and nerves pass. Inner enamel epithelium differentiate into ameloblasts which produce enamel prisms over the dentin (Fig. 13.9). The inner and outer enamel epithelia come together at the neck of the tooth to fold and form the epithelial root sheath, which grows into the mesenchyme and initiates root formation. The inner cells of the dental sac differentiate into cementoblasts, which

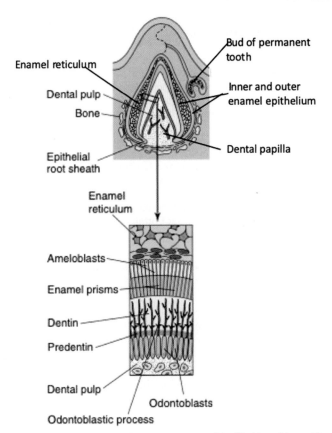

Fig. 13.9 Development of tooth structures. (Modified from Moore KL, Persaud TVN, Torchia MG. *The Developing Human: Clinically Oriented Embryology*. 10th ed. Philadelphia: Elsevier; 2015.)

produce cement that is restricted to the root. Cement is deposited over the dentin of the root and meets the enamel at the neck of the tooth.

- Eruption—As the root of the deciduous tooth grows, its crown gradually erupts through the oral epithelium with the oral mucosa around the crown becoming the gingiva. As permanent teeth grow, the root of the corresponding deciduous tooth is gradually resorbed by odontoclasts.

Molecular Biology Considerations

- BMP5, BMP7, GDF5, VEGF—chondrogenesis and skeletal development
- β-catenin levels, Runx2 and osterix (Osx), T-cell factor/lymphoid enhancer factor (TCF/LEF transcription factors) —osteogenesis, lineage commitment of skeletal precursor cells to chondrocytes and osteoblasts
- SOX9 and CARM1—regulation osteochondral ossification
- Wnt14, Noggin—early formation of the interzone
- Fat4 and Dchs1—early chondrogenesis in the vertebrae
- TBX6, HOX, PAX—regulate the patterning of the vertebrae along the anterior–posterior axis
- FGF10—induces formation of the apical ectodermal ridge
- BHLHA9, SHH—patterning of the limbs along the anterior–posterior axis.
- WNT7A, EN1—patterning the dorsal–ventral axis
- MYOD—induction of myogenesis in mesenchymal cells
- PBX, HAND2—cardiac muscle differentiation
- human TGF-β3—induction and morphogenesis of periodontal ligament
- TBX3, LEF1—formation of the mammary crests and buds.

CLINICAL ISSUES

LIMB ANOMALIES

If the development of the limb bud is suppressed early in the fourth week, amelia will result. If the disturbance occurs during the fifth week, a variant of meromelia will occur: – hemimelia, such as absence of the fibula in the leg; or phocomelia, in which the hands and/or feet are attached close to the body.

SPLIT-HAND/FOOT MALFORMATIONS

The failure of development of one or more digital rays results in the absence of one or more central digits. The hand or foot is divided into two parts that oppose and curve inward. This malformation originates during the fifth to sixth week of development.

OTHER ANOMALIES OF THE LIMBS AND DIGITS

- Symbrachydactyly—failure of the formation and differentiation of the axis of the entire limb including the hand plate. The thumb is often found coplanar to the hand.
- Polydactyly—supernumerary digits resulting from formation of additional digital rays.
- Cutaneous syndactyly—failure of the webs to degenerate between two or more digits.
- Osseous syndactyly—notches between the digital rays fail to form and develop and as a result, separation of the digits does not occur.
- Talipes equinovarus—a musculoskeletal deformation in which the sole of the foot is turned medially; the foot is inverted, preventing normal weight bearing.
- Developmental dysplasia of the hip—underdevelopment of the acetabulum and the head of the femur results in a joint capsule that is very relaxed, with dislocation almost always occurring after birth.
- Arthrogryposis—multiple congenital joint contractures and includes more than 300 heterogeneous disorders.

DEFECTS OF THE ABDOMINAL WALL

- Gastroschisis—a fissure in the abdominal wall, lateral to the median plane, resulting from failure of the lateral body walls to fuse. The bowel is uncovered and floats within the amniotic sac.
- Omphalocele—persistent herniation of the gut into the proximal umbilical cord, which results from hypoplasia of the muscle and skin of the abdominal wall.
- Prune belly syndrome—Abdominal muscle deficiency and hypotonia result in a thin abdominal wall. It is often associated with cryptorchidism and megaureters.

POLYMASTIA AND POLYTHELIA

An extra breast or nipple usually develops just inferior to the normal breast. This may occur in the axillary or abdominal regions and develop from extramammary buds that originate from remnants of the mammary crests. Supernumerary nipples in males may be mistaken for moles.

NUMERIC ABNORMALITY OF TOOTH NUMBERS

- Supernumerary teeth (mesiodens) usually develop near the maxillary incisors and can disrupt the position and eruption of normal teeth. The extra teeth commonly erupt posterior to the normal ones.
- Partial anodontia (one or more absent teeth); total anodontia is usually associated with ectodermal dysplasia.
- Macrodontia—partially divided tooth with a common root canal system.

Case Outcome

At birth, LE's baby had excess skin creases, brachydactyly, a depressed nasal bridge, a large head and shortened proximal limbs—typical features of achondroplasia.

Additional reflection: What features might be seen on a skeletal radiograph? What features might be found on genetic analysis and how do these findings correlate to the process of endochondral bone formation? The husband of LE is 47 years old; is this an important consideration? Why? If LE and her husband wish to have additional children, what considerations might be communicated to them? What might be the consequences of achondroplasia for a child, beyond short stature? How might achondroplasia impact adult health?

QUESTIONS

1. Ameloblasts produce which one of the following?
   a. Predentin
   b. Periodontal ligament
   c. Dentin
   d. Cementum
   e. Enamel

2. The majority of sebaceous glands develop as/from:
   a. downgrowth of the stratum germinativum
   b. hyperplasia of the epidermis
   c. buds from epidermal root sheath
   d. invagination of the surface ectoderm
   e. buds from preexisting eccrine sweat glands

3. Which of the following initiates the development of the limbs?
   a. Zone of polarising activity
   b. Endodermal cells at the apex of each limb bud
   c. Thoracic somites
   d. Proliferation of chondrocytes
   e. Apical ectodermal ridge

4. Myoblasts from the epaxial subdivision of cervical somites give rise to muscle in the:
   a. neck (extensors)
   b. tongue (intrinsic)
   c. eye (extrinsic muscles)
   d. face (muscles of expression)
   e. pharynx (constrictors)

5. Gastroschisis results from:
   a. persistent herniation of the gut into the umbilical cord
   b. failure of lateral body wall fusion
   c. abdominal muscle deficiency
   d. atresia of the foregut
   e. discordant positioning of the stomach

BIBLIOGRAPHY

I. Delgado, M. Torres, Coordination of limb development by crosstalk among axial patterning pathways, Dev Biol 429 (2017) 382–386.

R.J. Huebner, A.J. Ewald, Cellular foundation of mammary tubulogenesis, Semin Cell Dev Biol 31 (2014) 124–131.

N. Nandkishore, B. Vyas, A. Javali, et al. Divergent early mesoderm specification underlies distinct head and trunk muscle programmes in vertebrates, Development 145 (18) (2018)doi: 10.1242/dev.160945 pii: dev160945.

Y. Shi, B. Zhang, F. Kong, et al. Prenatal limb defects: epidemiologic characteristics and an epidemiologic analysis of risk factors, Medicine (Baltimore) 97 (29) (2018) e11471.

Teratogenesis and Birth Defects

14

Case Scenarios

Three cases for consideration:

- BB is a 48-year-old woman, pregnant with her first child, and attends her first prenatal visit at the start of her second trimester.
- OT is a 28-year-old woman who presents with a spontaneous abortion at approximately 6 weeks gestation. She used alcohol socially (2 ounces of alcohol per week) during weeks 1–4, before knowing that she was pregnant. She had since stopped drinking.
- GR is a 35-year-old woman recently immigrated to North America. Her only vaccinations have been for smallpox. GR wants to get pregnant. She appears to be considerably underweight. Her husband has a severe mobility issue, which you suspect may be as a result of untreated congenital hip dysplasia.

Questions for reflection: What risks do each of these cases present from the perspective of congenital anomalies? How might you counsel each woman?

In a majority of cases, the cause of birth defects is unknown; the remainder result from genetic or environmental factors, or are multifactorial inheritance with genes and the environment acting together. Most genetically abnormal embryos never become blastocysts and abort spontaneously with numeric or structural chromosomal abnormalities (Table 14.1).

The four clinically significant types of birth defects are:

- Malformation—morphological defect attributed to an intrinsically abnormal developmental process
- Disruption—morphological defect attributed to an extrinsic breakdown or interference with an originally normal developmental process
- Deformation—abnormal form, shape or position of a part of the body that results from mechanical forces
- Dysplasia—abnormal organisation of cells in tissues and the morphologic results.

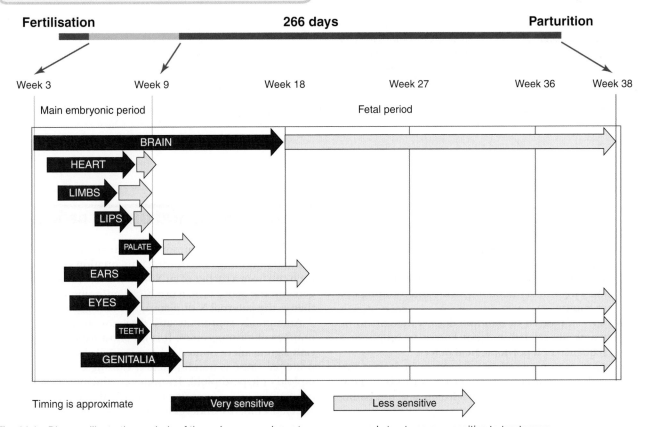

Fig. 14.1 Diagram illustrating periods of time when example systems, organs and structures are sensitive to teratogens.

Table 14.1   Incidence of select clinically relevant congenital anomalies

System	Condition	Reported Incidence (per 10,000 total births—live and stillbirths)
Neural tube defects	Anencephaly	1.2
	Spina bifida	3.2
	Encephalocele	0.8
Other central nervous system	Hydrocephaly	6.0
	Microcephaly	3.7
	Holoprosencephaly	0.8
Sense organs	Anophthalmia/microphthalmia	1.1
	Anotia/microtia	1.3
	Choanal atresia	2.7
Cardiac	Common truncus arteriosus	0.7
	Transposition of the great arteries	5.0
	Atrioventricular septal defect	4.6
	Tetralogy of Fallot	4.9
	Hypoplastic left heart syndrome	2.5
	Coarctation of the aorta	5.6
Orofacial clefts	Cleft palate only	6.0
	Cleft lip only	3.5
	Cleft lip with/without cleft palate	11.0
Alimentary system	Oesophageal atresia/tracheoesophageal fistula	2.8
	Small intestine atresia/stenosis	5.3
	Anorectal atresia/stenosis	3.4
Urinary system	Renal agenesis	3.9
	Cystic kidney disease	6.0
	Bladder and cloacal exstrophy	0.2
	Lower urinary tract obstruction	2.0
Genital system	Cryptorchidism	64.8
	Hypospadias	50.1
	Epispadias	2.0
	Indeterminate sex	1.7
Limbs	Limb deficiency defects	3.7
Body cavity	Diaphragmatic hernia	3.2
Abdominal wall defects	Omphalocele/exomphalos	2.0
	Gastroschisis	4.2
Chromosomal defects	Trisomy 21—Down syndrome	16.3
	Trisomy 13—Patau syndrome	1.2
	Trisomy 18—Edwards syndrome	2.6
	45,X—Turner syndrome	2.6

(From Public Health Infobase, Public Health Agency of Canada, Canadian Institute for Health Information – Discharge Abstract Database, 2005–2014.)

Other important concepts:

- Polytopic field defect—a pattern of defects derived from the disturbance of a single developmental field.
- Sequence—a pattern of multiple defects derived from a single known or presumed structural defect or mechanical factor. The primary initiating factor and resulting cascade are known.
- Syndrome—a pattern of multiple defects thought to be pathogenetically related and not known to represent a single sequence or a polytopic field defect.
- Association—the nonrandom occurrence in at least two individuals of multiple defects not known to be a polytopic field defect, sequence or syndrome, and not pathogenetically or causally related.

CHROMOSOMAL AND GENETIC DEFECTS

One of the two X chromosomes in female somatic cells may be randomly inactivated during implantation, and therefore each cell from a carrier of an X-linked disease has the mutant gene on the active or inactive X chromosome (expresses either as the paternal X or maternal X chromosome).

Aneuploidy represents any deviation from the diploid number of chromosomes. It is the most frequent and clinically significant of numeric chromosomal abnormalities; the principal cause is nondisjunction causing cells to be hypodiploid or hyperdiploid. Trisomies are the most frequent abnormalities of chromosome number, with more than 50% of affected embryos undergoing early spontaneous abortion.

The frequency of autosomal trisomy increases with maternal age. Sex chromosomal trisomy is more common than autosomal trisomy and the characteristic phenotype is not typically seen until puberty. Mosaicism occurs when an individual has at least two cell lines, with two or more genotypes, and it most commonly results in less serious defects than in those with monosomy or trisomy. If one oocyte is fertilised by two sperm or if there is failure of one meiotic division in a germ cell, triploidy will occur. Triploidy is usually fatal in the early neonatal period.

Structural chromosomal abnormalities include:

- translocation—transfer of a piece of one chromosome to a nonhomologous chromosome. A reciprocal translocation is found when two nonhomologous chromosomes exchange pieces of chromosome.
- deletion—loss of a part of a chromosome attributed to breakage. A ring chromosome occurs when there is a deletion at both ends of a chromosome and the broken ends rejoin.
- duplication—a duplicated part of a chromosome within a chromosome, attached to a chromosome, or a separate fragment.
- inversion—a segment of a chromosome is reversed; paracentric—confined to a single arm of the chromosome; pericentric—involves both arms and includes the centromere.
- isochromosome—when the centromere divides transversely a chromosome is created where one arm is missing and the other is duplicated.

Gene mutations cause about 8% of all birth defects and can result from environmental agents, such as ionising radiation. Such defects are inherited according to mendelian laws and probability of occurrence can be calculated. A comprehensive listing of all known human genetic disorders and gene loci can be found at the Online Mendelian Inheritance in Man (OMIM) website (www.ncbi.nlm.nih.gov/omim).

BIRTH DEFECTS CAUSED BY ENVIRONMENTAL FACTORS

Environmental teratogens cause 7% to 10% of birth defects; however, the exact mechanisms are generally unknown. Consideration of the teratogenicity of an agent requires consideration of the critical periods of development (peaks of cell division, differentiation and morphogenesis for the tissue, organ or system), dose of the teratogen (a dose relationship must be demonstrated for an environmental agent be considered a teratogen), and embryo genotype (there are genetic differences in response to a teratogen) (Table 14.2).

CLINICAL CONSIDERATIONS

TURNER SYNDROME

The most common chromosomal complement in Turner syndrome is 45,X; however, about 50% of individuals with Turner syndrome have other karyotypes. Only 1% of affected embryos survive. The phenotype is female, but without hormone replacement the majority of individuals do not develop secondary sex characteristics. Other phenotypic characteristics include a webbed neck, prominent ears, short stature, widely spaced nipples with broad chest and lymphoedema in the hands and feet.

TRISOMY 21—DOWN SYNDROME

The chromosomal complement in Down syndrome is 47,XX, + 21 or 47,XY, + 21, resulting from nondisjunction (most frequently in the mother). The incidence of trisomy 21 increases with maternal age. In almost all cases the individuals have both cognitive and physical disabilities. Phenotypic characteristics include brachycephaly, slanted palpebral fissures, flat nasal bridge, macroglossia, transverse palmar flexion crease, congenital heart defects, umbilical hernia and reduced muscle tone.

PRADER-WILLI AND ANGELMAN SYNDROMES

These are typically associated with deletion of band q12 on chromosome 15, and the phenotype is determined by the parental origin of the defective chromosome. The origin of Prader-Willi syndrome is the father's chromosome; the phenotype is characterised by hypotonia, poor growth and delayed development, and in adulthood hyperphagia attributed to insatiable appetite starting in childhood, underdeveloped genitalia and infertility. Angelman syndrome originates from the mother's chromosome, with the phenotype characterised by microcephaly, macrosomia, delayed development, ataxia, hyperactivity, cognitive disabilities, seizures and scoliosis.

FRAGILE X SYNDROME

This is the most commonly known inherited cause of intellectual disability and one of more than 200 X-linked disorders associated with mental impairment. Fragile X syndrome is the result of an expansion of CGG nucleotides in *FMR1* gene, typically repeated more than 200 times. Males are usually more affected that females, with characteristics including intellectual disability, anxiety and hyperactivity, and with some individuals having autism spectrum disorder.

EXAMPLES OF TERATOGEN EFFECTS

ALCOHOL

Neonates born to mothers with chronic alcoholism demonstrate growth deficiency, mental deficiency, microcephaly, short palpebral fissures, maxillary hypoplasia, joint defects, congenital heart disease and other birth defects. Fetal alcohol spectrum disorder is the preferred term for the range of prenatal alcohol effects. There is no known safe level for alcohol consumption during pregnancy. Moreover, the susceptible period of brain development spans the major part of gestation and as such total abstinence from alcohol during pregnancy is recommended.

ISOTRETINOIN

Isotretinoin (13-*cis*-retinoic acid) is used for treating severe cystic acne. The critical period appears to be from

Table 14.2   Common known human teratogens

Teratogen	Most Common Birth Defects
Drugs	
Alcohol	Fetal alcohol syndrome: IUGR, mental deficiency, microcephaly, ocular anomalies, joint abnormalities, short palpebral fissures
Androgens and high doses of progestogens	Masculinisation of female fetuses: ambiguous external genitalia
Aminopterin	IUGR; skeletal defects; CNS malformations, notably meroencephaly
Carbamazepine	Neural tube defects, craniofacial defects, developmental retardation
Cocaine	IUGR, prematurity, microcephaly, cerebral infarction, urogenital defects, neurobehavioral disturbances
Diethylstilboestrol	Abnormalities of uterus and vagina
Isotretinoin (13-*cis*-retinoic acid)	Craniofacial abnormalities, neural tube defects, cardiovascular defects, cleft palate, thymic aplasia
Lithium carbonate	Defects of the heart and great vessels
Methotrexate	Skeletal defects involving the face, cranium, limbs and vertebral column
Misoprostol	Limb abnormalities, ocular and cranial nerve defects, autism spectrum disorder
Phenytoin	Fetal hydantoin syndrome
Tetracycline	Stained teeth, hypoplasia of enamel
Thalidomide	Meromelia, amelia, facial defects, cardiac, kidney and ocular defects
Trimethadione	Development delay, V-shaped eyebrows, low-set ears, cleft lip and/or palate
Valproic acid	Craniofacial anomalies, neural tube defects, cognitive abnormalities, often hydrocephalus, heart and skeletal defects
Warfarin	Nasal hypoplasia, stippled epiphyses, hypoplastic phalanges, eye anomalies, mental deficiency
Chemicals	
Methylmercury	Cerebral atrophy, spasticity, seizures, mental deficiency
Polychlorinated biphenyls	IUGR, skin discoloration
Infections	
Cytomegalovirus	Microcephaly, chorioretinitis, sensorineural hearing loss, delayed psychomotor/mental development, hepatosplenomegaly, hydrocephaly, cerebral palsy, periventricular (brain) calcification
Hepatitis B virus	Preterm birth, low birth weight, fetal macrosomia
Herpes simplex virus	Skin vesicles and scarring, chorioretinitis, hepatomegaly, thrombocytopenia, petechiae, haemolytic anaemia, hydranencephaly
Human parvovirus B19	Fetal anaemia, nonimmune hydrops fetalis, fetal death
Rubella virus	IUGR, postnatal growth retardation, cardiac and great vessel abnormalities, microcephaly, sensorineural deafness, cataract, microphthalmos, glaucoma, pigmented retinopathy, mental deficiency, neonate bleeding, hepatosplenomegaly, osteopathy, tooth defects
Toxoplasma gondii	Microcephaly, mental deficiency, microphthalmia, hydrocephaly, chorioretinitis, cerebral calcifications, hearing loss, neurological disturbance
Treponema pallidum	Hydrocephalus, congenital deafness, mental deficiency, abnormal teeth and bones
Venezuelan equine encephalitis virus	Microcephaly, microphthalmia, cerebral agenesis, CNS necrosis, hydrocephalus
Zika virus	Microcephaly, neurological disorders, retinal mottling, macular degeneration, contractures, hypotonia.
Varicella virus	Cutaneous scars, limb paresis, hydrocephaly, seizures, cataracts, microphthalmia, Horner syndrome, optic atrophy, nystagmus, chorioretinitis, microcephaly, mental deficiency, limb and digit hypoplasia, urogenital anomalies
Radiation	
High levels of ionising radiation	Microcephaly, mental deficiency, skeletal anomalies, growth retardation, cataracts

CNS, Central nervous system; *IUGR,* intrauterine growth retardation.

week 3 to 5. The most common major defects present in affected infants are craniofacial dysmorphism, microtia, micrognathia, cleft palate, thymic aplasia, cardiovascular defects, neural tube defects and neuropsychological impairment.

RUBELLA VIRUS

Maternal infection with the rubella virus in the first trimester results in congenital rubella syndrome, features of which include cataracts, cardiac defects and deafness, and in some cases, intellectual deficiency, glaucoma, microphthalmia and tooth defects. Maternal infection in the second and third trimesters may result in intellectual deficiency and hearing loss.

Case Outcomes

Follow-up for the cases:

- BB—amniocentesis demonstrated a karyotype of 46,XX/47,XX, + 21.
- OT—presents 6 months later and 4 weeks pregnant, and is concerned about the risk of a second spontaneous abortion as a result of her taking aspirin (600 mg, every 6 hours, for 2 days) for a headache, before recognising she was pregnant.
- GR—refused vaccination in spite of your discussion. She has now returned to the clinic with symptoms of rubella infection; she has just reached her third trimester.

Additional reflection: What risks do each of these cases present from the perspective of congenital anomalies? How might you counsel each woman?

QUESTIONS

1. In teratology, a syndrome would be defined as:
   a. a pattern of defects derived from a disturbance of a single developmental field
   b. a morphological defect attributed to extrinsic breakdown of an originally normal process
   c. a pattern of multiple defects not known to be from a single sequence
   d. the abnormal formation of a body part resulting from mechanical forces
   e. a pattern of multiple defects derived from a single defect or factor

2. Which of the following is correct regarding Turner syndrome?
   a. A majority of embryos with Turner syndrome survive
   b. The most common chromosomal compliment is 45,X
   c. The phenotype is male, but secondary sex characteristics do not develop
   d. The phenotype is female and secondary sex characteristics develop without pharmaceutical intervention
   e. The most common chromosomal compliment is 47,XX, + 21

3. Deletion of band q15 on chromosome 15 results in:
   a. Prader-Willi syndrome if the parental original of the defect is the mother

   b. hyperphagia if the parental original of the defect is the father
   c. Angelman syndrome if the parental original of the defect is the father
   d. microcephaly if the parental original of the defect is the father
   e. scoliosis if the parental original of the defect is the father

BIBLIOGRAPHY

Baldacci S, Gorini F, Santoro M, et al. Environmental and individual exposure and the risk of congenital anomalies: a review of recent epidemiological evidence. Epidemiol Prev 2018;42(3–4 Suppl 1):1–34.

Burd L, Popova S. Fetal alcohol spectrum disorders: fixing our aim to aim for the fix. Int J Environ Res Public Health 2019;16:3978.

Foeller ME, Lyell DJ. Marijuana use in pregnancy: concerns in an evolving era. J Midwifery Womens Health 2017;62:363–7.

Goncalves LF, Lee W, Mody S, et al. Diagnostic accuracy of ultrasonography and magnetic resonance imaging for the detection of fetal anomalies: a blinded case-control study. Ultrasound Obstet Gynecol 2016;48:185–92.

Hill MA. Two web resource linking human embryology collections worldwide. Cells Tissues Organs 2018;205:293–302.

Mejdoubi M, Monthieux A, Cassan T, et al. Brain MRI in infants after maternal Zika virus infection during pregnancy. N Engl J Med 2017;14.

Wagner R, Tse WH, Gosemann JH, et al. Prenatal maternal biomarkers for the early diagnosis of congenital malformations: a review. Pediatr Res 2019;doi: 10.1038/s41390-019-0429-1.

Multiple Choice Question Answers

CHAPTER 2—REPRODUCTIVE ORGANS AND GAMETOGENESIS

1. Answer: C. Spermatids do not divide. They are gradually transformed into mature sperm during spermiogenesis.
2. Answer: B. Trisomy is a relatively common numerical chromosomal anomaly resulting from an error in meiotic cell division during gametogenesis. When homologous chromosomes fail to separate and migrate to opposite poles of the germ cell, some gametes have 24 chromosomes and others have 22. This abnormal condition is known as nondisjunction. In the event of fertilisation occurring between a gamete with 24 chromosomes and a normal gamete with 23 chromosomes, the resulting zygote has 47 chromosomes (trisomy). Spermatogonia are the primitive male germ cells with a chromosomal constitution of 46,XY, and they give rise to the spermatozoa. Spermatids differentiate into mature spermatozoa by a process known as spermiogenesis.

CHAPTER 3—FERTILISATION AND REPRODUCTIVE TECHNOLOGIES

1. Answer: D. Typically 300 million sperms are deposited in the vagina during sexual intercourse. Usually 200 million to 600 million sperms are in the ejaculate, but only a few hundred sperms are believed to reach the fertilisation site. If less than 50 million sperms are present in a semen sample, the male from whom the sample was taken may be infertile.
2. Answer: C. When a sperm contacts the cell membrane of a secondary oocyte, the oocyte completes the second maturation or meiotic division and becomes a mature ovum or oocyte. The second polar body, a nonfunctional cell, is formed during this division. If fertilisation does not occur, the secondary oocyte does not complete this division; it degenerates within 24 hours after ovulation.
3. Answer: B. The sperm digests a path through the corona radiata and zona pellucida by the action of enzymes, including hyaluronidase, released from the sperm's acrosome through perforations that develop in it during the acrosome reaction. Tubal mucosal enzymes appear to assist hyaluronidase. Movements of the tail of the sperm are also involved in this process.
4. Answer: E. It is believed that structurally abnormal sperm do not fertilise ova because of their lack of normal motility and fertilising ability. Examination of semen is important in the study of fertility. The number, motility, and abnormalities in size and shape of sperm are important in assessing sterility in males. If 20% or more sperm are morphologically abnormal, fertility usually is impaired.

CHAPTER 4—IMPLANTATION AND WEEK 2

1. Answer: B. The trophoblast is composed of the cytotrophoblast and the syncytiotrophoblast. The amniotic sac and umbilical vesicle are contained within the chorionic cavity.
2. Answer: B. The amniotic cavity is found between the trophoblast and the epiblast, a component of the inner cell mass. The chorion envelops the amniotic sac. The connecting stalk is invested with amnion and is the precursor to the umbilical cord.
3. Answer E. Ectopic pregnancies in locations other than the ampulla of the uterine tube are rare. A cervical pregnancy is not considered ectopic (outside the uterus) but is abnormal.
4. Answer: A. Partial hydatidiform moles are typically dispermic. In both types of mole, the embryo is absent, but the trophoblast proliferates. Affected women present with vomiting, vaginal bleeding and an enlarging uterus. Less that 5% of molar pregnancies develop into a choriocarcinoma, a highly metastatic cancer.

CHAPTER 5—WEEKS 3 TO 8 AND GENERAL ORGANOGENESIS

1. Answer: C. The primitive streak is the first morphological sign of gastrulation. The primitive pit forms by proliferation of the cranial end of the streak, whereas the primitive groove develops as a furrow in the streak. Cells from the hypoblast and primitive streak displace hypoblast cells to form the endoderm.
2. Answer: D. The notochord induces the formation of neuroepithelium, which forms the neural plate and folds. Neural tube closure begins at approximately day 21. The neural crest cells are highly mobile.

CHAPTER 6—PLACENTATION AND MEMBRANES

1. Answer: B. Monochorionic twins result from division of the blastocyst or embryoblast, are identical and share one chorionic sac.
2. Answer: C. After 11 to 14 weeks, trophoblastic cell plugs in the spiral arteries disintegrate, resulting in an increase in oxygen concentrations. The intervillous space contains maternal blood. The placenta is initially formed of syncytiotrophoblast, cytotrophoblast, villous connective tissue, and endothelium of the fetal vessels. By the start of week 8, chorionic villi associated with the decidua capsularis become compressed and necrotic, leading to a smooth portion of the chorion.

3. Answer: A. The placenta synthesises glycogen, oestrogen and glucose, the latter of which is transported by facilitated diffusion (GLUT1). In the placenta, oxygenation is flow limited.

4. Answer: D. Preeclampsia often includes proteinuria, and may include reduced liver or renal function, thrombocytopenia and pulmonary oedema. Placenta previa results from implantation adjacent to the internal uterine os and may cause bright red bleeding after about 20 weeks. Fetal erythroblastosis is not related to ABO incompatibility, but may include other antigen incompatibilities beyond Rh, such as Xg, Cc and Kell. Twin transfusion syndrome is most common in monochorionic–diamniotic monozygotic twins.

CHAPTER 7—FETAL AND NEONATAL PERIODS

1. Answer: E. Labour comprises cervical dilation, expulsion and the placental stage. Oxytocin and relaxin are produced by the mother to elicit uterine contractions and impact cervical dilation, respectively. Contractions increase in intensity and occur more frequently as the cervix dilates.

2. Answer: D. The transition from fetal to neonatal life happens very rapidly. For instance, fluid from the lungs is cleared quickly through the lymphatic system. Only about 10% of infants require some minor assistance to begin breathing, with fewer than 1% requiring resuscitation. Delayed clamping of the cord is now included in many clinical guidelines and has been shown to increase haemoglobin and iron stores.

3. Answer: B. Intrauterine growth retardation (IUGR) can result from fetal, maternal, placental or environmental causes, and depending on the timing of the impact of those factors, the fetus may show either a symmetric or asymmetric pattern of IUGR. Ongoing fetal ultrasound is important once IUGR is suspected, to monitor growth changes. Infants with a history of IUGR have an increased risk of neurological and cognitive issues.

CHAPTER 8—CARDIOVASCULAR, HAEMATOPOIETIC AND LYMPHATIC SYSTEMS

1. Answer: C. The septum secundum contributes to the closure of the foramen secundum. The primordial pulmonary vein contributes to the formation of most of the wall of the left atrium.

2. Answer: A. The umbilical veins carry highly oxygenated blood. The ductus venosus develops and shunts about one-half of the blood from the left umbilical vein around the liver and directly to the heart. The superior vena cava develops from the right anterior and common cardinal veins, whereas the inferior vena cava has four segments, derived from several sources.

3. Answer: A. The ductus arteriosus has a physiological sphincter to prevent overloading of the heart. The ductus arteriosus and foramen ovale close quickly after birth, but do not attain anatomical closure for about 3 months.

4. Answer: B. Although ventricular septal defect (VSD) is the most common septation defect at birth, 30% to 50% of the defects close without treatment by 1 year of age. The most common cardiac anomaly in trisomy 21 is endocardial cushion defect with ostium primum atrium septum defect (ASD). Tetralogy of Fallot may or may not result in cyanosis.

CHAPTER 9—BODY CAVITIES, RESPIRATORY, DIAPHRAGM, AND HEAD AND NECK

1. Answer: D. The thyroid (as well as cricoid and arytenoid) arches are derived from the fourth and sixth pharyngeal arches. The fifth pharyngeal arch is rudimentary. Epiglottal cartilage is derived from the hypobranchial eminence (from the third and fourth pharyngeal arches).

2. Answer: C. These secondary clefts extend through the soft and hard palates and are posterior to the incisive fossa. Primary palate clefts result from lack of fusion of the palatine processes with the mesenchyme derived from the medial nasal prominences form the primary palate.

3. Answer: C. At approximately 24 weeks, which is the beginning of the terminal sac stage.

4. Answer: A. Contents from the abdominal cavity within the thoracic cavity restrict lung growth. CHAOS results in hyperinflated lungs, whereas respiratory distress syndrome results from reduced surfactant production in the lungs. A tracheoesophageal fistula occurs with incomplete fusion of the tracheoesophageal folds. First arch syndrome presents with defects of the ears, mandible, palate or eyes, resulting from reduced neural crest cell migration.

5. Answer: D. Initially, the septum transversum develops from the ventrolateral body wall, and is imbedded with a large portion of the liver. Later, as folding occurs, the septum transversum fuses with the pleuroperitoneal membranes and the dorsal mesentery of the oesophagus, forming a partial partition between the abdominal and thoracic cavities.

CHAPTER 10—NERVOUS SYSTEM, EYES, EARS

1. Answer: C. The double-layered, pigmented epithelium of the iris develops from the inner and outer layers of the rim of the optic cup. Because this epithelium is continuous with the ciliary epithelium and the retina, it often is wrongly assumed to be homologous only to the pigmented layers of these structures derived from the outer layer of the optic cup.

2. Answer: C. Atresia of the external acoustic meatus canal is a relatively common condition. It often is unilateral and associated with abnormalities of the auricle. Failure of the meatal plug of the first pharyngeal groove to canalise leads to atresia of the external acoustic meatus. This anomaly usually results from autosomal dominant inheritance.

3. Answer: E. The neurons that form the grey matter in the ventral (anterior) horns of the spinal cord are derived from neuroblasts in the basal plates. The lateral grey columns of the spinal cord are also derived from the basal plates. The alar laminae form the grey columns in the dorsal horns.

4. Answer: E. The walls of the metencephalon give rise to the pons and cerebellum; its cavity forms the superior part of the fourth ventricle.

CHAPTER 11—ALIMENTARY SYSTEM

1. Answer: E. The celiac artery arises from the anterior aspect of the aorta inferior to the aortic hiatus. It subdivides into left gastric, hepatic and splenic arteries that supply almost all of the foregut derivatives. The superior and inferior mesenteric arteries supply the mid- and hindgut respectively. Intersegmental arteries provide blood to the somites from the dorsal aorta.
2. Answer: B. The pectinate line is found at the inferior border of the anal valves. The blood and nerve supplies to the areas inferior and superior to the pectinate line differ. For instance, inferior to the pectinate line, the anal canal is supplied by somatic sensory cutaneous fibres. The levator ani forms the largest portion of the pelvic floor. The urorectal septum divides the cloaca to separate the hindgut from the urinary system.
3. Answer: D. In anorectal agenesis, the rectum ends superior to the puborectalis muscle, the latter being the demarcation between high and low anomalies. Anorectal agenesis is often associated with fistula including rectourethral fistulae. Imperforate rectum (a low anorectal anomaly) describes the anal canal ending blindly.
4. Answer: A. Both the ventral and dorsal pancreatic buds form from endodermal cells of the foregut. The uncinate process and part of the head of the pancreas are formed from the ventral pancreatic bud. The pancreas begins to secrete insulin by 10 weeks, although glucagon is secreted a few weeks later. An annular pancreas can remain asymptomatic until adulthood, when signs of duodenal obstruction may occur with pancreatitis.

CHAPTER 12—UROGENITAL SYSTEM

1. Answer: C. Primordial germ cells will be found located between the endoderm and mesoderm of the umbilical vesicle, near the origin of the allantois. The primordial germ cells then migrate along the dorsal mesentery, into the gonadal ridges and incorporated into the primary sex cords.
2. Answer: E. The ureteric bud is an outpouch of the mesonephric duct, adjacent to the junction of the duct with the urogenital sinus. The paramesonephric duct forms from mesothelium of the mesonephric duct and is an important contributor to the female reproductive system. Intermediate mesoderm is the source of cells for the nephrogenic cord, the origin of the urogenital system.
3. Answer: A. The uterus develops by the fusion of the paramesonephric ducts and the degeneration of the intervening septum. The mesonephric duct does not play a significant role in the development of the female reproductive system. The sinovaginal bulbs fuse to form the vaginal plate. The urogenital sinus, derived from division of the cloaca by the urorectal septum, forms structures including the bladder and urethra.
4. Answer: E. In ovotesticular disorder of sexual differentiation (DSD), the individual has both testicular and ovarian tissue (either as an ovotestis or separately), and the external genitalia are ambiguous. Sex chromosome DSD results from nondisjunction of the sex chromosome during meiosis. Congenital adrenal hyperplasia results from a defect in the synthesis pathway of adrenal steroids. In androgen sensitivity syndrome, testosterone is produced, but there is a resistance to the effects of testosterone at the cellular level. Potter sequence results from reduced amniotic fluid volume, subsequent compression of the fetus, deformations such as depressed nasal bridge, and pulmonary hypoplasia because of chest wall compression.

CHAPTER 13—SKELETAL, MUSCLE AND INTEGUMENT

1. Answer: E. The ameloblasts differentiate from the inner enamel epithelium and produce enamel prisms over the dentin. Mesenchymal cells in the dental papilla differentiate into odontoblasts which produce predentin. Predentin calcifies to become dentin. Neural crest cells differentiate to form the periodontal ligament.
2. Answer: C. Eccrine sweat glands develop as buds from the epidermis whereas apocrine seat glands develop from the stratum germinativum.
3. Answer: E. The apical ectodermal ridge develops from ectodermal cells at the apex of each limb bud location and initiates development. The limb buds develop opposite caudal cervical segments. The zone of polarising activity helps to control anterior–posterior axis orientation. As the limbs develop, chondrification appears by about week 5 to form the bone models.
4. Answer: A. Epaxial myoblasts give rise to the extensor muscles of the neck. The others are formed from:
   • intrinsic muscles of the tongue—occipital myotomes
   • extrinsic muscles of the eye—preotic myotomes
   • muscles of facial expression—second pharyngeal arch
   • pharyngeal constrictors—fourth arch.
5. Answer: B. An omphalocele results from persistent herniation whereas prune belly syndrome results from muscle deficiency.

CHAPTER 14—TERATOGENESIS AND BIRTH DEFECTS

1. Answer: C.
   Answer A describes a polytopic field defect. Answer B describes a disruption. Answer D describes a deformation, while answer E describes a sequence.
2. Answer: B. Only about 1% of embryos with 45,X survive. The phenotype is female but without hormone replacement, secondary sex characteristics do not develop. Phenotypic characteristics include a webbed neck and lymphoedema in the hands and feet, as opposed to individuals with trisomy 21 (47,XX, + 21 or 47,XY, + 21) who characteristically have brachycephaly, macroglossia and reduced muscle tone.
3. Answer: B. Prader-Willi syndrome results when the defect arises from the father and the phenotype includes hyperphagia. Angelman syndrome occurs when the defect arises from the mother and the phenotype includes microcephaly and scoliosis.

Index

Page numbers followed by "*f*" indicate figures, "*t*" indicate tables, and "*b*" indicate boxes.